Colorectal Cancer

Editor

LEONARD B. SALTZ

HEMATOLOGY/ONCOLOGY CLINICS OF NORTH AMERICA

www.hemonc.theclinics.com

Consulting Editors
GEORGE P. CANELLOS
H. FRANKLIN BUNN

February 2015 • Volume 29 • Number 1

ELSEVIER

1600 John F. Kennedy Boulevard • Suite 1800 • Philadelphia, Pennsylvania, 19103-2899

http://www.theclinics.com

HEMATOLOGY/ONCOLOGY CLINICS OF NORTH AMERICA Volume 29, Number 1
February 2015 ISSN 0889-8588, ISBN 13: 978-0-323-32652-0

Editor: Jessica McCool
Developmental Editor: Donald Mumford

Hematology/Oncology Clinics (ISSN 0889-8588) is published bimonthly by Elsevier Inc., 360 Park Avenue South, New York, NY 10010-1710. Months of issue are February, April, June, August, October, and December. Business and Editorial Offices: 1600 John F. Kennedy Blvd., Ste. 1800, Philadelphia, PA 19103—2899. Customer Service Office: 3251 Riverport Lane, Maryland Heights, MO 63043. Periodicals postage paid at New York, NY and at additional mailing offices. Subscription prices are $385.00 per year (domestic individuals), $633.00 per year (domestic institutions), $190.00 per year (domestic students/residents), $440.00 per year (Canadian individuals), $783.00 per year (Canadian institutions) $520.00 per year (international individuals), $783.00 per year (international institutions), and $255.00 per year (international and Canadian students/residents). International air speed delivery is included in all *Clinics* subscription prices. All prices are subject to change without notice. **POSTMASTER:** Send address changes to *Hematology/Oncology Clinics of North America*, Elsevier Health Sciences Division, Subscription Customer Service, 3251 Riverport Lane, Maryland Heights, MO 63043. Customer Service (orders, claims, online, change of address): Elsevier Health Sciences Division, Subscription Customer Service, 3251 Riverport Lane, Maryland Heights, MO 63043. Tel: 1-800-654-2452 (U.S. and Canada); 314-447-8871 (outside U.S. and Canada). Fax: 314-447-8029. E-mail: journalscustomerservice-usa@elsevier.com (for print support); journalsonlinesupport-usa@elsevier.com (for online support).

Reprints. For copies of 100 or more, of articles in this publication, please contact the Commercial Reprints Department, Elsevier Inc., 360 Park Avenue South, New York, New York 10010-1710; Tel.: 212-633-3874, Fax: 212-633-3820, E-mail: reprints@elsevier.com.

Hematology/Oncology Clinics of North America is covered in *MEDLINE/PubMed (Index Medicus), EMBASE/ Excerpta Medica, and BIOSIS.*

Contributors

CONSULTING EDITORS

GEORGE P. CANELLOS, MD
William Rosenberg Professor of Medicine; Department of Medical Oncology, Dana-Farber
Cancer Institute, Boston, Massachusetts

H. FRANKLIN BUNN, MD
Professor of Medicine; Division of Hematology, Brigham and Women's Hospital,
Harvard Medical School, Boston, Massachusetts

EDITOR

LEONARD B. SALTZ, MD
Professor of Medicine, Weill Cornell Medical College; Chief, Gastrointestinal Oncology
Service, Department of Medicine, Memorial Sloan Kettering Cancer Center, New York,
New York

AUTHORS

EMILY K. BERGSLAND, MD
Professor of Clinical Medicine, UCSF Helen Diller Family Comprehensive Cancer Center,
San Francisco, California

CARLOS H.F. CHAN, MD, PhD
Division of Surgical Oncology, Massachusetts General Hospital Cancer Center, Boston,
Massachusetts

JAMES C. CUSACK, MD
Division of Surgical Oncology, Massachusetts General Hospital Cancer Center, Boston,
Massachusetts

MICHAEL I. D'ANGELICA, MD, FACS
Enid A. Haupt Chair in Surgery; Attending Surgeon, Hepatopancreatobiliary Service,
Memorial Sloan Kettering Cancer Center; Associate Professor, Cornell University Weill
Medical College, New York, New York

ANGELITA HABR-GAMA, MD, PhD
Professor of Surgery, Angelita and Joaquim Gama Institute; University of São Paulo
School of Medicine, São Paulo, Brazil

JUSTIN Y. JEON, PhD
Professor, Exercise Medicine Center for Cancer and Diabetes Patients, Department of
Sport and Leisure Studies, Yonsei University, Seoul, Korea

JUNGA LEE, PhD
Postdoctoral Research Fellow, Exercise Medicine Center for Cancer and Diabetes
Patients, Department of Sport and Leisure Studies, Yonsei University, Seoul, Korea

HEINZ-JOSEF LENZ, MD
Sharon Carpenter Laboratory, University of Southern California/Norris Comprehensive Cancer Center, Keck School of Medicine, Los Angeles, California

JEFFREY A. MEYERHARDT, MD, MPH
Associate Professor of Medicine, Department of Medical Oncology, Dana-Farber Cancer Institute, Boston, Massachusetts

RODRIGO O. PEREZ, MD, PhD
Angelita and Joaquim Gama Institute; Colorectal Surgery Division, Department of Gastroenterology, University of São Paulo School of Medicine, São Paulo, Brazil

ELENA N. PETRE, MD
Research Scientist, Memorial Sloan Kettering Cancer Center, New York, New York

DAVID P. RYAN, MD
Division of Medical Oncology, Massachusetts General Hospital Cancer Center, Boston, Massachusetts

GUILHERME PAGIN SÃO JULIÃO, MD
Angelita & Joaquim Gama Institute, Paraiso, São Paulo, Brazil

ANA SEBIO, MD
Sharon Carpenter Laboratory, University of Southern California/Norris Comprehensive Cancer Center, Keck School of Medicine, Los Angeles, California

J. JOSHUA SMITH, MD, PhD
Surgical Oncology Fellow, Department of Surgery, Memorial Sloan Kettering Cancer Center, New York, New York

CONSTANTINOS T. SOFOCLEOUS, MD, PhD
Assistant Professor, Memorial Sloan Kettering Cancer Center, New York, New York

STEPHEN B. SOLOMON, MD
Professor, Memorial Sloan Kettering Cancer Center, New York, New York

ZSOFIA K. STADLER, MD
Assistant Attending Physician, Clinical Genetics and Gastrointestinal Oncology Services, Department of Medicine, Memorial Sloan Kettering Cancer Center; Assistant Professor of Medicine, Department of Medicine, Weill Cornell Medical College, New York, New York

SEBASTIAN STINTZING, MD
Sharon Carpenter Laboratory, University of Southern California/Norris Comprehensive Cancer Center, Keck School of Medicine, Los Angeles, California; Department of Hematology and Oncology, University of Munich, Munich Germany

STEFAN STREMITZER, MD
Sharon Carpenter Laboratory, University of Southern California/Norris Comprehensive Cancer Center, Keck School of Medicine, Los Angeles, California

Contents

patients with a complete clinical response who could possibly be managed nonoperatively with strict follow-up (watch-and-wait strategy). The present article deals with critical issues regarding appropriate selection of patients for this approach.

A Critical Look at Local-Regional Management of Peritoneal Metastasis

Carlos H.F. Chan, James C. Cusack, and David P. Ryan

For patients with stage IV colorectal cancer, the presence of peritoneal metastases is a poor prognostic feature. Despite the improvement in systemic therapy, long-term survival remains poor for patients with peritoneal carcinomatosis. Cytoreductive surgery (CRS) and hyperthermic intraperitoneal chemotherapy (HIPEC) can be associated with long-term survival in patients who have limited peritoneal disease, particularly those who can have complete cytoreduction. Whether the possible benefit of CRS and HIPEC is from the surgical resection of all disease or the combination of CRS and HIPEC remains unclear.

HEMATOLOGY/ONCOLOGY CLINICS OF NORTH AMERICA

FORTHCOMING ISSUES

April 2015
Bladder Cancer
Joaquim Bellmunt, *Editor*

June 2015
Complement-mediated Hemolytic Anemias
Robert A. Brodsky, *Editor*

August 2015
Pancreatic Cancer
Brian Wolpin, *Editor*

RECENT ISSUES

December 2014
Bone Marrow Transplantation
Bipin N. Savani and Mohamad Mohty, *Editors*

October 2014
Multiple Myeloma
Kenneth C. Anderson, *Editor*

August 2014
Iron Disorders
Matthew M. Heeney and Alan R. Cohen, *Editors*

ISSUE OF RELATED INTEREST

Surgical Oncology Clinics of North America, January 2014 (Vol. 23, Issue 1)
Treatment of Colorectal Cancer
Nancy N. Baxter and Marcus J. Burnstein, MD
Available at: http://www.surgonc.theclinics.com/

VISIT THE CLINICS ONLINE!
Access your subscription at:
www.theclinics.com

NOW AVAILABLE FOR YOUR iPhone and iPad

Preface

Colorectal Cancer

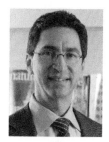

Leonard B. Saltz, MD
Editor

The management of colorectal cancer has evolved dramatically over the past several decades and continues to do so. Despite widespread agreement on many aspects of this disease, many controversies still remain. The nature of medical or scientific situations in which controversies remain between informed individuals is that the data are insufficient, or insufficiently compelling, to allow for a clear definitive "one right answer" that would be acceptable to all. For this reason, the articles contained within this issue, which are all written by bona fide experts in the field, often espouse opinions and interpretations of available data that are, at least to some degree, in conflict with one another. This should not be interpreted as either inconsistency or the presence of some "right" and some "wrong" opinions, but rather, as a reflection of the state-of-the-art, in which multiple reasonable interpretations of the data and so, multiple reasonable courses of action, are available to us. Consideration of all of these interpretations, and individualization of management as a result, is now the coin of the realm.

I thank the authors for their outstanding and thoughtful contributions, and I hope the readers will find these articles as stimulating, thought-provoking, and helpful as I have, in refining my thoughts and approach to both the clinical and the research aspects of the management of the patient with colorectal cancer.

Leonard B. Saltz, MD
Memorial Sloan Kettering Cancer Center
300 East 66th Street
New York, NY 10065, USA

E-mail address:
saltzl@MSKCC.ORG

Hematol Oncol Clin N Am 29 (2015) ix
http://dx.doi.org/10.1016/j.hoc.2014.10.012
0889-8588/15/$ – see front matter © 2015 Elsevier Inc. All rights reserved.

Diet and Lifestyle in Survivors of Colorectal Cancer

Junga Lee, PhD[a], Justin Y. Jeon, PhD[a],
Jeffrey A. Meyerhardt, MD, MPH[b],*

KEYWORDS

- Colorectal cancer • Cancer survival • Lifestyle factors • Epigenetics

KEY POINTS

- Lifestyle factors that include obesity, physical activity, and diet are emerging as potential critical elements in improving survival outcomes for colorectal cancer.
- Changes in individual health behaviors both before and after a diagnosis of colorectal cancer may improve outcomes of survivors.
- Studies have indicated that maintaining a normal weight, participating in regular physical activity, and eating a healthy diet may be important preventive steps leading to improved survival outcomes.
- Epigenetic studies have demonstrated, at the cellular level, the possible mechanisms of colorectal cancer that can be positively influenced by changing lifestyle.

INTRODUCTION

The American Cancer Society estimates that there are more than 1.1 million survivors of colorectal cancer in the United States.[1] Survivors of colorectal cancer constitute 10% of the total number of cancer survivors, and the number is increasing.[2] Both genetic and lifestyle factors contribute to cancer development and the prognosis of colorectal cancer. Because lifestyle factors such as obesity, physical inactivity, diet, smoking, and alcohol consumption are potentially modifiable[3,4] while genetic factors are not, much attention has been paid to the impact of lifestyle factors on the incidence and prognosis of colorectal cancer.

Changing these modifiable factors toward practice of a healthy lifestyle may be crucial components of cancer treatment in addition to standard treatments in preventing recurrence and improving survival of patients with colorectal cancer. Although an increasing number of studies have examined the association of diet and lifestyle

[a] Exercise Medicine Center for Cancer and Diabetes Patients, Department of Sport and Leisure Studies, 50 Yonsei-ro, Yonsei University, Seoul 120-749, Korea; [b] Department of Medical Oncology, Dana-Farber Cancer Institute, 450 Brookline Avenue, Boston, MA 02215, USA
* Corresponding author.
E-mail address: jmeyerhardt@partners.org

Hematol Oncol Clin N Am 29 (2015) 1–27
http://dx.doi.org/10.1016/j.hoc.2014.09.005
0889-8588/15/$ – see front matter © 2015 Elsevier Inc. All rights reserved.
hemonc.theclinics.com

factors with cancer recurrence and survival outcome in patients with locally advanced colorectal cancer,[5–9] it is important to distinguish whether these exposures were measured before or after cancer diagnosis. For example, adiposity before diagnosis and after diagnosis may have a different impact on survival outcomes of patients with colorectal cancer. Exposures after diagnosis associated with prognosis of cancer may provide important implications on directing recommendations to cancer survivors. However, if an association exists only between prediagnosis adiposity and prognosis of colorectal cancer, it is less certain how to guide a patient, although such data may be important in understanding the biology of colorectal cancer.

This review summarizes the associations of modifiable lifestyle factors, including prediagnosis and postdiagnosis adiposity, physical activity, and diet, on the prognosis of patients with colorectal cancer. Given that most published data to date are from patients without metastatic disease, the focus here is on associations of these factors in survivors of stage I to III colorectal cancer. This article also summarizes the possible mechanisms for the association between modifiable lifestyle factors and the prognosis of patients with colorectal cancer.

ASSOCIATION BETWEEN THE PREDIAGNOSIS LIFESTYLE FACTORS AND RISK OF MORTALITY IN SURVIVORS OF COLORECTAL CANCER

Adiposity

Several studies have examined the association between prediagnosis adiposity and the prognosis of colorectal cancer (**Table 1**).[6,10–13] These studies used a variety of metrics for adiposity, including body mass index (BMI; calculated as weight in kilograms divided by height in meters squared, ie, kg/m^2), waist-hip ratio (WHR), and waist circumference (WC). Campbell and colleagues[6] examined 2303 men and women with stage I to III colorectal cancer and reported that those with BMI higher than 25 had worse colorectal cancer–specific mortality and all-cause mortality. Similarly, Doria-Rose and colleagues[10] studied 633 postmenopausal women with colorectal cancer and reported that obese patients (BMI $\geq$30) had a 2.1-fold higher risk of colorectal cancer–specific mortality and all-cause mortality compared with patients of normal weight.

Other studies have reported similar findings when using alternative measurements for adiposity such as percent body fat, WC, and WHR. Haydon and colleagues[14] reported that patients with colorectal cancer with increasing WC per 10 cm had a 1.33-times higher risk of disease-specific death. The investigators concluded that prediagnosis abdominal obesity might be a critical risk factor for mortality in patients with all-cause mortality, and made the recommendation for maintaining a normal weight and WC. In a study that compared BMI, weight, WHR, and WC, Prizment and colleagues[11] reported that whereas higher BMI ($\geq$25) and weight ($\geq$63.5 kg) were not significantly associated with colon cancer mortality, higher WHR ($\geq$0.81) and WC ($\geq$82.5 cm) were significantly associated with mortality. This study suggested that WHR and WC, which reflect abdominal adiposity, might be better predictors of colon cancer mortality than BMI and weight.

Physical Activity

Reports on association between the level of physical activity before cancer diagnosis and the risk of mortality in patients with colorectal cancer have been mixed (**Table 2**).[12,14–17] Some studies found significant associations between level of prediagnosis physical activity levels[12,14] and the risk of mortality, whereas others have found no association.[15] Meyerhardt and colleagues[15] studied female patients with stage I to III colorectal cancer and did not find any association between the level of prediagnosis physical activity and the risk of mortality. On the other hand, Haydon and colleagues[14] found that prediagnosis physical activity level was significantly associated with increased disease-specific survival. The authors have recently performed a meta-analysis of the association between prediagnosis physical activity and the risk of mortality in patients with stage I to III colorectal cancer.[7] The meta-analysis demonstrated that patients with colorectal cancer who participated in any amount of physical activity exhibited 25% and 24% risk reduction in colorectal cancer–specific death and death from all causes, respectively, compared with patients who did not participate in any physical activity. The study also found a dose-dependent risk reduction in colorectal cancer–specific death and all-cause death, suggesting that those who participated in more physical activity before diagnosis have a lower risk of recurrence and death after the completion of standard therapy.

Diet

Diverse dietary factors are related to the development of colorectal cancer,[18] yet few studies have focused on diet before diagnosis and mortality for patients with colorectal cancer (**Table 3**).[8,19,20] Among the diverse dietary factors, there is relatively consistent evidence that red and processed meat is related to an increased risk of colorectal cancer.[21] Recently, McCullough and colleagues[8] collected diet information from 2315 participants diagnosed with colorectal cancer in 1992/1993, 1999, and 2003, and followed their mortality through December 31, 2010. Those with higher red and processed meat intake (fourth quartile) before cancer diagnosis were reported to have a 29% and 63% increase in all-cause and cardiovascular disease mortality, respectively, compared with those with low red and processed meat intake (first quartile). An association between the amount of red and processed meat intake and colorectal cancer–specific mortality was not observed. Furthermore, Zell and colleagues[19] studied 511 patients with colorectal cancer (144 familial and 376 sporadic colorectal cancer), and found that those who had high meat intake had reduced 10-year overall survival (4th quartile 42% vs 1st–3rd quartile 65%) and a 2.24-times increased risk of death in an adjusted analysis compared with those who had low meat intake among familial patients with colorectal cancer. No association was observed between the amount of meat intake and overall survival in sporadic patients with colorectal cancer. In addition, Zhu and colleagues[20] performed a 1-year recall of meat intake in 529 survivors of colorectal cancer and reported that the highest quartile of processed meat intake was significantly associated with poorer disease-free survival (hazard ratio [HR] 1.82, 95% confidence interval [CI] 1.07–3.09) and overall survival (HR 2.13, 95% CI 1.03–4.43) in patients with colon cancer. However, they did not observe any significant association between the amount of processed meat intake and survivor outcomes in patients with rectal cancer. Furthermore, they found no associations between prudent vegetable or the high-sugar pattern and disease-free and overall survival in patients with colon and rectal cancer.

Mechanism for Prediagnosis Energy Balance Factors and Outcomes

Several hypotheses on why energy balance–associated host factors before diagnosis may negatively affect the prognosis of colorectal cancer have been proposed. First, many patients who have unfavorable energy balance (ie, obese or physically inactive) before diagnosis will be in a similar situation after diagnosis. Obesity and physical inactivity are associated with insulin resistance and subsequent hyperinsulinemia, which is linked to increased risk for cancer and mortality because it induces insulin-like growth factors (IGFs) that promote cancer growth.[22] Patients with colorectal

Table 1
Prospective cohort studies of prediagnosis body mass index (BMI, kg/m^2) and survival outcomes in patients with colorectal cancer

Authors,[Ref.] Year, Name of Cohort, Country	Study Participants	Median Years of Follow-Up	Relative Risk/Hazard Ratio (95% Confidence Interval)		Adjustment Factors
Doria-Rose, et al,[10] 2006, Wisconsin Cancer Reporting System, USA	633 female Colon and rectal	9.4	**CRC-specific mortality**		Age, stage, postmenopausal hormone use, and smoking
			<20.0	1.6 (0.9–3.1)	
			20.0–24.9	Referent	
			25.0–29.9	1.3 (0.9–1.9)	
			≥30	1.5 (0.9–2.6)	
			All-cause mortality		
			<20.0	1.5 (1.0–2.4)	
			20.0–24.9	Referent	
			25.0–29.9	1.2 (0.9–1.6)	
			≥30	1.5 (1.0–2.2)	
Prizment et al,[11] 2010, Iowa Women's Health Study, USA	1096 female Colon	20	**CRC-specific mortality**		Stage, age, education, and smoking
			<18.5	1.84 (0.84–4.03)	
			18.5–24.9	Referent	
			25.0–29.9	1.18 (0.87–1.52)	
			≥30	1.35 (1.00–1.82)	
			All-cause mortality		
			<18.5	1.89 (1.01–3.53)	
			18.5–24.9	Referent	
			25.0–29.9	1.12 (0.89–1.41)	
			≥30	1.45 (1.14–1.85)	
Kuiper et al,[12] 2012, Women's Health Initiative, USA	1339 female Colon and rectal	11.9	**CRC-specific mortality**		Age, study arm, BMI, tumor stage, ethnicity, education, alcohol, smoking, hormone therapy use
			18.5–24.9	Referent	
			25.0–29.9	0.77 (0.52–1.13)	
			≥30	1.17 (0.80–1.72)	
			All-cause mortality		
			18.5–24.9	Referent	
			25.0–29.9	0.90 (0.66–1.23)	
			≥30	1.19 (0.88–1.62)	

Campbell et al,[6] 2012, Cancer Prevention Study-II Nutrition Cohort, USA	2303 both genders Colon and rectal	16		Age, sex, smoking status, BMI, red meat intake, tumor stage, leisure time spent sitting, education
			CRC-specific mortality	
			Female	
			<18.5	0.83 (0.25–2.76)
			18.5.0–24.9	Referent
			25.0–29.9	1.19 (0.80–1.78)
			≥30	1.52 (0.96–2.41)
			Male	
			<18.5	Not reported
			18.5.0–24.9	Referent
			25.0–29.9	1.06 (0.77–1.48)
			≥30	1.31 (0.88–1.95)
			Both	
			<18.5	0.67 (0.21–2.12)
			18.5.0–24.9	Referent
			25.0–29.9	1.09 (0.85–1.40)
			≥30	1.35 (1.01–1.80)
			All-cause mortality	
			Female	
			<18.5	1.74 (0.85–3.58)
			18.5.0–24.9	Referent
			25.0–29.9	1.22 (0.95–1.63)
			≥30	1.42 (1.01–2.00)
			Male	
			<18.5	1.40 (0.55–3.56)
			18.5.0–24.9	Referent
			25.0–29.9	0.97 (0.79–1.19)
			≥30	1.21 (0.94–1.57)
			Both	
			<18.5	1.53 (0.88–2.66)
			18.5.0–24.9	Referent
			25.0–29.9	1.06 (0.90–1.25)
			≥30	1.30 (1.06–1.58)

(continued on next page)

Table 1
(continued)

Authors,[Ref.] Year, Name of Cohort, Country	Study Participants	Median Years of Follow-Up	Relative Risk/Hazard Ratio (95% Confidence Interval)	Adjustment Factors
Pelser et al,[13] 2014, NIH-AARP Diet and Health Study, USA	4213 colon 1514 rectal Both genders	5	**CRC-specific mortality among colon cancer cases**	Lag time, sex, education, family history of colon cancer, cancer stage, first course of treatment (surgery, radiation, chemotherapy), and also mutually adjusted for quintiles of HEI-2005 scores, BMI, physical activity, alcohol, and smoking history
			18.5–24.9 Referent	
			25.0–29.9 0.97 (0.82–1.15)	
			≥30 1.15 (0.96–1.39)	
			All-cause mortality	
			18.5–24.9 Referent	
			25.0–29.9 1.02 (0.88–1.17)	
			≥30 1.19 (1.02–1.39)	
			CRC-specific mortality among rectal cancer cases	
			18.5–24.9 Referent	
			25.0–29.9 0.92 (0.70–1.22)	
			≥30 1.04 (0.75–1.44)	
			All-cause mortality	
			18.5–24.9 Referent	
			25.0–29.9 0.85 (0.68–1.07)	
			≥30 1.00 (0.77–1.30)	

cancer with higher levels of C-peptide (a breakdown product of insulin production at the time of diagnosis) have shown higher mortality compared with those who had lower levels of C-peptide.[23] Also, these host factors induce an increasing level of tumor necrosis factor (TNF)-α, interleukin (IL)-6, or leptin that promotes cancer growth, along with a decreasing level of adiponectin that also promotes cancer growth.[24–29] Given that the primary risk for patients with stage I to III colorectal cancer is growth of occult micrometastases, such growth factors can stimulate micrometastases that lead to recurrent disease.

Prediagnosis obesity or physical inactivity may affect the molecular nature of the colorectal cancer that develops, leading to more aggressive histology. For example, obesity and physical inactivity are associated with the development of CTNNB1 (β-catenin)-negative colorectal cancer.[30] CTNNB1 tumors have a trend toward worse colorectal cancer–specific survival.[31] In obese patients, nuclear CTNNB1 negativity was associated with significantly worse cancer-specific and overall survival. Similarly, among patients with nuclear CTNNB1-negative stage I to III, postdiagnosis physical activity was associated with significantly better cancer-specific survival, whereas physical activity was not associated with survival among patients with nuclear CTNNB1-positive stage I to III.

In terms of red and processed meat and survival, prior research has indicated that several factors may be instrumental in cancer development. Such factors include: (1) production of heterocyclic amines when meat is cooked at high temperature[32]; (2) involvement of N-nitroso compounds from the heme in the gastrointestinal tract[33,34]; and (3) use of nitrosamines, N-nitroso compounds, and their precursors, owing to nitrite or nitrate use in the preservation of meat.[35] However, it is unclear if increased exposure to these factors will lead to more aggressive cancers.

ASSOCIATION BETWEEN POSTDIAGNOSIS LIFESTYLE FACTORS AND THE RISK OF MORTALITY
Adiposity

Reports on postdiagnosis BMI and outcomes in colorectal cancer have been mixed (**Table 4**).[5,6,12,36–41] Some studies showed that being obese may have a negative impact on the survival of colorectal cancer,[6,36,37,41] whereas other studies showed that there is no association between postdiagnosis obesity and the prognosis of colorectal cancer.[38] In one early report, Meyerhardt and colleagues[36] examined the association between obesity and prognosis of patients with stage II and III colon cancer, and found that female patients with a BMI of 30 or greater were associated with a 34% significant increase in mortality and a 24% nonstatistically significant increase in disease recurrence, whereas there was no such association between obesity and disease recurrence in men. Dignam and colleagues[37] reported on a similar population of patients with colon cancer, and found a statistically significant 38% increase in the risk of recurrence and 28% increase in the risk of mortality among patients with a BMI greater than or equal to 35, and did not find an interaction by gender. One study, limited to patients with rectal cancer, did not show any significant association between BMI and disease-free or overall survival,[38] although subgroup analyses by Campbell and colleagues[6] did suggest that obesity was associated with worse outcomes in patients with rectal cancer.

In studying the impact of being obese after diagnosis of colorectal cancer on its prognosis, it is very important to consider reverse causality, meaning that less obese patients may have worse prognosis if the reason for lower body weight might well be related to disease progression.[42] Some people have lower body mass as a result of a

Table 2
Prospective cohort studies of prediagnosis physical activity and survival outcomes in patients with colorectal cancer

Authors,[Ref.] Year, Name of Cohort, Country	Study Participants	Median Years of Follow-Up	Relative Risk/Hazard Ratio (95% Confidence Interval)		Adjustment Factors
Haydon et al,[14] 2006, Melbourne Collaborative Cohort Study, Australia	526 both genders Colon and rectal	5.5	**CRC-specific mortality** Exerciser vs nonexerciser	0.73 (0.54–1.00)	Age, sex, stage, BMI
			All-cause mortality Exerciser vs nonexerciser	0.77 (0.58–1.03)	
Meyerhardt et al,[15] 2006, Nurses' Health Study, USA	573 female Colon and rectal	9.6	**CRC-specific mortality** *<3 MET-h/wk* *3–8.9* *9–17.9* *≥18*	Referent 0.83 (0.45–1.53) 1.05 (0.56–1.99) 0.86 (0.44–1.67)	Age, stage, tumor differentiation, year of diagnosis, time between study entry to questionnaire, BMI, smoking
			All-cause mortality *<3 MET-h/wk* *9–8.9* *9–17.9* *≥18*	Referent 0.85 (0.52–1.37) 1.14 (0.69–1.87) 0.95 (0.57–1.59)	
Meyerhardt et al,[16] 2009, Health Professionals Follow-up Study, USA	599 male Colon and rectal	8.6	**CRC-specific mortality** *<3 MET-h/wk* *3.1–9.0* *9.1–18* *18.1–27* *≥27*	Referent 0.56 (0.28–1.13) 0.64 (0.33–1.24) 0.53 (0.26–1.10) 0.52 (0.29–0.94)	Age, stage, year of diagnosis, tumor differentiation, tumor location, BMI, smoking
			All-cause mortality *<3 MET-h/wk* *3.1–9.0* *9.1–18* *18.1–27* *≥27*	Referent 0.55 (0.36–0.85) 0.60 (0.41–0.89) 0.51 (0.34–0.79) 0.48 (0.34–0.69)	

Study	N, cancer type	MET-h/wk	Outcome	HR (95% CI)	Adjustments
Kuiper et al,[12] 2012, Women's Health Initiative, USA	1339 female Colon and rectal	11.9	**CRC-specific mortality**		Age, study arm, BMI, tumor stage, ethnicity, education, alcohol, smoking, hormone therapy use
			0 MET-h/wk	*Referent*	
			>0–2.9	0.98 (0.58–1.66)	
			3.0–8.9	1.01 (0.65–1.57)	
			9.0–17.9	0.74 (0.46–1.20)	
			≥18.0	0.68 (0.41–1.13)	
			All-cause mortality		
			0 MET-h/wk	*Referent*	
			>0–2.9	0.93 (0.61–1.43)	
			3.0–8.9	1.01 (0.71–1.43)	
			9.0–17.9	0.77 (0.52–1.12)	
			≥18.0	0.63 (0.42–0.96)	
Campbell et al,[17] 2013, Cancer Prevention Study-II, USA	2262 both genders Colon and rectal	6.8	**CRC-specific mortality**		Age, sex, smoking status, BMI, red meat intake, tumor stage, leisure time spent sitting, education
			<3.5 MET-h/wk	*Referent*	
			3.5–<8.75	0.68 (0.49–0.95)	
			≥8.75	0.78 (0.57–1.08)	
			All-cause mortality		
			<3.5 MET-h/wk	*Referent*	
			3.5–<8.75	0.69 (0.55–0.85)	
			≥8.75	0.72 (0.58–0.89)	

Abbreviation: MET-h/wk, metabolic-equivalent task hours per week.

Table 3
Prospective cohort studies of prediagnosis diet and survival outcomes in patients with colorectal cancer

Authors,[Ref.] Year, Name of Cohort, Country	Study Participants	Median Years of Follow-Up	Dietary Measure	Relative Risk/Hazard Ratio (95% Confidence Interval)		Adjustment Factors
Zell et al,[19] 2006, USA	511 both genders Colon and rectal	7.9	Red and processed meat	**All-cause mortality** Quartiles 1–3 vs Quartiles 4	Familial CRC; 2.24 (1.25–4.03) Sporadic CRC; 1.02 (0.67–1.15)	Age, stage, and sex
Zhu et al,[20] 2013, Newfoundland Familial Colorectal Cancer Registry, Canada	529 both genders Colon and rectal	6.4	Processed meat dietary pattern	**Disease-free survival** Highest vs lowest quartile	1.82 (1.07–3.09)	Total energy intake, sex, age at diagnosis, stage at diagnosis, marital status, family history, reported screening procedure, reported chemoradiotherapy and microsatellite instability status, where appropriate.
McCullough et al,[8] 2013, Cancer Prevention Study-II Nutrition Cohort, USA	2315 both genders Colon and rectal	7.5	Red and processed meat	**All-cause mortality** Top vs bottom quartile	1.29 (1.05–1.59)	Age at diagnosis, sex, tumor stage at diagnosis, 1992 energy intake

Abbreviation: CRC, colorectal cancer.

Table 4
Prospective cohort studies of postdiagnosis BMI and survival outcomes in patients with colorectal cancer

Authors,[Ref.] Year, Name of Cohort, Country	Study Participants	Median Years of Follow-Up	Relative Risk/Hazard Ratio (95% Confidence Interval)		Adjustment Factors
Meyerhardt et al,[36] 2003, National Cancer Institute INT-0089, USA	3759 both genders Colon	9.4	**All-cause mortality**		Age, race, baseline, performance status, bowel obstruction, bowel perforation, Duke stage, presence of peritoneal implants, predominant macroscopic pathologic feature, and completion chemotherapy
			Female		
			<21	1.08 (0.87–1.35)	
			21–24.9	Referent	
			25.0–27.49	1.18 (0.94–1.49)	
			27.5–29.9	1.23 (0.95–1.60)	
			≥30	1.34 (1.07–1.67)	
			Male		
			<21	1.33 (1.05–1.67)	
			21–24.9	Referent	
			25.0–27.49	1.03 (0.87–1.22)	
			27.5–29.9	0.96 (0.78–1.17)	
			≥30	0.94 (0.77–1.15)	
			Both		
			<21	1.15 (0.98–1.35)	
			21–24.9	Referent	
			25.0–27.49	1.10 (0.95–1.26)	
			27.5–29.9	1.05 (0.90–1.24)	
			≥30	1.11 (0.96–1.29)	

(continued on next page)

Table 4
(continued)

Authors,[Ref.] Year, Name of Cohort, Country	Study Participants	Median Years of Follow-Up	Relative Risk/Hazard Ratio (95% Confidence Interval)		Adjustment Factors
Meyerhardt et al,[53] 2004, National Cancer Institute INT-0114, USA	1688 Both genders Rectal	9.9	**All-cause mortality**		Age, race, nodal status, extent of tumor invasion, clinical bowel obstruction, and distance from anal verge
			Female		
			<21	1.29 (0.87–1.91)	
			21–24.9	Referent	
			25.0–27.49	0.75 (0.49–1.16)	
			27.5–29.9	0.89 (0.61–1.33)	
			≥30	0.94 (0.66–1.33)	
			Male		
			<21	1.62 (1.08–2.43)	
			21–24.9	Referent	
			25.0–27.49	1.07 (0.86–1.33)	
			27.5–29.9	0.99 (0.79–1.25)	
			≥30	1.19 (0.94–1.52)	
			Both		
			<21	1.43 (1.08–1.89)	
			21–24.9	Referent	
			25.0–27.49	0.97 (0.80–1.17)	
			27.5–29.9	0.95 (0.78–1.15)	
			≥30	1.09 (0.9–1.33)	

Dignam et al,[37] 2006, National Surgical Adjuvant Breast and Bowel Project Randomized Trials, USA	4288 Female Colon	11.2	**All-cause mortality** <21.0 21.0–24.9 25.0–29.9 30–34.9 ≥30	1.49 (1.17–1.91) Referent 1.02 (0.91–1.14) 1.11 (0.96–1.28) 1.28 (1.04–1.57)	Age, sex, race, performance status, number of positive lymph nodes, presence of bowel obstruction, and treatment
Meyerhardt et al,[38] 2008, National Cancer Institute CALGB 89803, USA	1053 both genders Colon	5.3	**All-cause mortality** <21.0 21.0–24.9 25.0–29.9 30–34.9 ≥30	1.07 (0.61–1.87) Referent 0.72 (0.50–1.03) 0.90 (0.61–1.34) 0.87 (0.54–1.42)	Sex, age, depth of invasion through bowel wall, number of positive lymph node, presence of clinical perforation at time of surgery, presence of bowel obstruction, baseline carcinoembryonic antigen, grade of tumor differentiation, baseline performance status, treatment arm, weight change between first and second questionnaire, BMI at the time or second questionnaire, and time between study entry and completion of second questionnaire

(continued on next page)

Table 4
(continued)

Authors,[Ref.] Year, Name of Cohort, Country	Study Participants	Median Years of Follow-Up	Relative Risk/Hazard Ratio (95% Confidence Interval)		Adjustment Factors
Sinicrope et al,[39] 2010, ACCENT Group database, USA	4381 both genders Colon	8	**All-cause mortality**		Age, stage, treatment, and sex
			Female		
			<20.0	1.32 (1.05–1.67)	
			20.0–24.9	Referent	
			25.0–29.9	1.18 (0.94–1.49)	
			30–34.9	1.24 (1.01–1.53)	
			≥30	1.11 (0.84–1.45)	
			Male		
			<20.0	1.14 (0.81–1.61)	
			20.0–24.9	Referent	
			25.0–29.9	0.82 (0.71–0.95)	
			30–34.9	0.94 (0.78–1.15)	
			≥30	1.35 (1.02–1.79)	
			Both		
			<20.0	1.24 (1.03–1.5)	
			20.0–24.9	Referent	
			25.0–29.9	0.90 (0.80–1.00)	
			30–34.9	1.07 (0.93–1.23)	
			≥30	1.19 (0.98–1.45)	
Baade et al,[5] 2011, Queensland, Australia	2561 both genders Colon and rectal	4.9	**CRC-specific mortality**		Age, sex, stage at diagnosis, smoking, site of tumor, treatment (surgery only vs surgery and adjuvant therapy)
			<18.5	1.74 (0.85, 3.58)	
			18.5.0–24.9	Referent	
			25.0–29.9	0.75 (0.59–0.97)	
			≥30	1.34 (0.70–2.58)	
			Unknown	1.34 (0.70–2.58)	
			All-cause mortality		
			<18.5	2.29 (1.47–3.59)	
			18.5.0–24.9	Referent	
			25.0–29.9	0.75 (0.61–0.94)	
			≥30	0.78 (0.59–1.03)	
			Unknown	0.94 (0.51–1.74)	

Study	Population	Follow-up (y)	Outcome / BMI category	HR (95% CI)	Covariates
Chin et al,[40] 2012, China	2765 both genders Colon and rectal	5	**CRC-specific mortality**		Tumor, nodes, metastasis stage, age, gender, comorbidities, carcinoembryonic antigen, hemoglobin, albumin, operative timing, postoperative morbidity, tumor location, histologic type, and histologic grade
			Female		
			<18.5	1.16 (0.75–1.82)	
			18.5.0–24.9	Referent	
			25.0–29.9	0.96 (0.60–1.43)	
			≥30	1.11 (0.84–1.43)	
			Male		
			<18.5	1.46 (0.84–2.52)	
			18.5.0–24.9	Referent	
			25.0–29.9	0.96 (0.69–1.32)	
			≥30	1.21 (0.83–1.77)	
			Both		
			<18.5	1.33 (0.94–1.87)	
			18.5.0–24.9	Referent	
			25.0–29.9	0.96 (0.76–1.2)	
			≥30	1.06 (0.80–1.41)	
			All-cause mortality		
			Female		
			<18.5	1.55 (1.11–2.16)	
			18.5.0–24.9	Referent	
			25.0–29.9	0.95 (0.71–1.27)	
			≥30	0.99 (0.69–1.41)	
			Male		
			<18.5	1.55 (1.03–2.35)	
			18.5.0–24.9	Referent	
			25.0–29.9	0.77 (0.58–1.01)	
			≥30	0.91 (0.66–1.25)	
			Both		
			<18.5	1.58 (1.23–2.05)	
			18.5.0–24.9	Referent	
			25.0–29.9	0.83 (0.68–1.01)	
			≥30	0.94 (0.68–1.01)	
Kuiper et al,[12] 2012, Women's Health Initiative, USA	676 Female Colon and rectal	11.9	**CRC-specific mortality**		Age, study arm, time from diagnosis to measurement, prediagnostic BMI, tumor stage, ethnicity, education, alcohol, smoking, hormone therapy use
			18.5.0–24.9	Referent	
			25.0–29.9	0.45 (0.22–0.92)	
			≥30	0.95 (0.49–1.85)	
			All-cause mortality		
			18.5.0–24.9	Referent	
			25.0–29.9	0.78 (0.47–1.27)	
			≥30	1.09 (0.65–1.83)	

(continued on next page)

Table 4
(continued)

Authors,[Ref.] Year, Name of Cohort, Country	Study Participants	Median Years of Follow-Up	Relative Risk/Hazard Ratio (95% Confidence Interval)		Adjustment Factors
Campbell et al,[17] 2013, Cancer Prevention Study-II Nutrition Cohort, USA	2303 both genders Colon and rectal	6.8	**CRC-specific mortality**		Age, sex, smoking status, BMI, red meat intake, tumor stage, leisure time spent sitting, education
			Female		
			<18.5	0.39 (0.12–1.32)	
			18.5.0–24.9	Referent	
			25.0–29.9	0.81 (0.50, 1.31)	
			≥30	1.09 (0.60, 2.01)	
			Male		
			<18.5	2.48 (0.55–11.3)	
			18.5.0–24.9	Referent	
			25.0–29.9	0.91 (0.61–1.34)	
			≥30	1.29 (0.82–2.01)	
			Both		
			<18.5	0.64 (0.25–1.60)	
			18.5.0–24.9	Referent	
			25.0–29.9	0.87 (0.65–1.17)	
			≥30	1.14 (0.81–1.60)	
			All-cause mortality vs BMI		
			Female		
			<18.5	1.19 (0.65–2.18)	
			18.5.0–24.9	Referent	
			25.0–29.9	0.84 (0.60–1.16)	
			≥30	1.19 (0.79–1.78)	
			Male		
			<18.5	2.78 (1.29–5.96)	
			18.5.0–24.9	Referent	
			25.0–29.9	0.82 (0.66–1.03)	
			≥30	0.89 (0.67–1.18)	
			Both		
			<18.5	1.30 (0.82–2.06)	
			18.5.0–24.9	Referent	
			25.0–29.9	0.83 (0.70–1.00)	
			≥30	0.93 (0.75–1.17)	

Sincrope et al,[41] 2013, National Cancer Institute and conducted by Mayo Clinic/North Central Cancer Treatment Group and the Southwest Oncology group, USA	25291 both genders Colon	7.8	**All-cause mortality**	Age, stage, treatment, and sex
			Female	
			<20.0	1.12 (1.00–1.25)
			20.0–24.9	Referent
			25.0–29.9	1.05 (0.97–1.14)
			30–34.9	1.10 (0.99–1.23)
			≥35	1.07 (0.93–1.24)
			Male	
			<20.0	1.39 (1.21–1.60)
			20.0–24.9	Referent
			25.0–29.9	0.95 (0.87–1.02)
			30–34.9	1.10 (1.99–1.2)
			≥35	1.16 (1.0–1.35)
			Both	
			<20.0	1.21 (1.11–1.32)
			20.0–24.9	Referent
			25.0–29.9	1.10 (1.04–1.17)
			30–34.9	1.10 (1.02–1.18)
			≥35	1.11 (1.00–1.23)

healthy lifestyle including exercise and diet while some people lose weight as a result of cancer recurrence. This concept may be one of the reasons why postdiagnosis obesity seems to associate less with prognosis of colorectal cancer in comparison with prediagnosis obesity; this is the limitation of observational epidemiologic studies. In addition, nearly all studies to date have focused on BMI because of the availability of height and weight in these cohort studies. However, other measures of adiposity may be more appropriate and should be considered in future studies. Finally, even if a certain level of adiposity is associated with worse outcomes, it is unclear as to whether changing weight would influence this association. Only one study to date has reported the impact of weight change after diagnosis on the prognosis of patients with colon cancer. Meyerhardt and colleagues[38] studied weight gain or weight loss from approximately 3 months after surgery to approximately 15 months after surgery in patients with stage III colon cancer, and found no significant associations with either gain or loss for cancer recurrences or mortality. Ultimately, randomized controlled trials of weight control and reduction would be needed to further understand such a relationship.

Physical Activity

Studies of the association between postdiagnosis physical activity and the risk of recurrence and mortality in patients with colorectal cancer have led to fairly consistent conclusions (**Table 5**).[5,12,15–17,43] An increasing level of physical activity significantly improved overall mortality in patients with colorectal cancer and either significantly or nonsignificantly trended to improved disease-free survival or colorectal cancer–specific mortality. In a recent meta-analysis of prospective cohort studies,[7] the authors found that patients with any physical activity after diagnosis had reduced risk of colorectal cancer–specific mortality (relative risk [RR] 0.74, 95% CI 0.58–0.95), compared with patients with no physical activity. Those who participated in high levels of physical activity after diagnosis (vs low levels) had an RR of 0.65 (95% CI 0.47–0.92). Although efforts in these studies are made to account for potential for reverse causality, one cannot fully eliminate the potential that ability to be more active may be reflective of a healthier survivor of colorectal cancer. Furthermore, whether increasing the level of physical activity after diagnosis will improve outcome is unknown at this time.

Diet

As was found with prediagnosis diet and colorectal mortality, few studies have examined the association between postdiagnosis diet and mortality for patients with colorectal cancer (**Table 6**).[8,9,44] In contrast to their prior study of prediagnosis patients, McCullough and colleagues[8] reported that red and processed meat intake after diagnosis was not independently associated with survival outcomes. On the other hand, Meyerhardt and colleagues[9] reported an association between Western dietary pattern, which consisted of red and processed meat, refined grains, and sugar desserts, and the risk of recurrence and mortality in patients with colon cancer. Meyerhardt and colleagues[9] studied 1009 patients with colon cancer, and collected dietary information within 3 months of surgery (while on adjuvant therapy) and 6 months after completing adjuvant chemotherapy. Using cumulative averaging of these 2 dietary time points and factor analysis to determine dietary patterns, the investigators found that the highest quintile in the Western dietary pattern group had a 3.25-times worse disease-free survival compared with the lowest quintile. In a second study of the same cohort of patients, patients with the highest quintile of glycemic load had a 1.79-times higher risk of recurrence and morality compared with the lowest quintile.[44] Interestingly the association between glycemic load and outcomes was influenced by

BMI ($P_{interaction}$ =.01). Whereas glycemic load was not associated with disease-free survival in patients with BMI less than 25, higher glycemic load was statistically significantly associated with worse disease-free survival among overweight or obese participants (BMI $\geq$25; HR 2.26, 95% CI 1.53–3.32). This interaction further supports the potential relationship between energy balance and outcomes in patients with colorectal cancer.

Mechanism for Postdiagnosis Energy Balance Factors and Outcomes

For patients with nonmetastatic colorectal cancer at the time of diagnosis, the primary risk within the first several years is recurrence of disease. Recurrences are presumed to be micrometastases in primarily distant organs that over time grow to become detectable metastases. The presumed role of adjuvant therapy is to combat these micrometastases, whether through direct cell death or other mechanisms. It is not known if all micrometastases will grow to manifest as frank recurrences. However, several factors are presumed to help stimulate cell growth, including insulin and insulin-related growth factors. Obesity, lack of physical activity, Western pattern diet, and high glycemic load are known to increase insulin resistance, which increases the level of insulin. Given that insulin is one of the most potent apoptosis inhibitors and that an insulin-reducing agent metformin inhibits cancer cell proliferation,[45,46] these factors leading to unfavorable energy balance can induce hyperinsulinemia and increase the risk of recurrence by stimulating the growth of micrometastases. Furthermore, hyperinsulinemia increases the production of IGF-1, which is another cell growth factor. These negative energy balance factors can increase adipocytokines (leptin and adiponectin), as discussed earlier.[28] An exercise intervention was found to reduce leptin, TNF-α, and IL-6, while increasing adiponectin levels, for patients with colorectal cancer.[47]

Independent of risk of recurrences of colorectal cancer, hyperinsulinemia patients may be more vulnerable to other diseases such as type 2 diabetes and cardiovascular disease, which is one of best known causes of mortality in patients with colorectal cancer.[6] Furthermore, during cancer treatment various clinical and molecular factors including chemotherapy, other treatments, and drugs could alter vulnerability and lead to inflammation and pathogenesis for those patients with colorectal cancer who are obese, thereby reducing survivorship.[48]

Recent molecular epidemiology studies have further strengthened the potential mechanism for energy balance and outcomes. For patients with colon cancer who had CDKN1B (p27) expression (a potent cyclin-dependent kinase inhibitor), at least 18 metabolic-equivalent task hours (MET-hours) per week physical activity was associated with 67% in colon cancer–specific mortality, compared with less than 18 MET-hours per week.[16] For patients with CDKN1B loss, there was no association between physical activity and mortality outcome. This finding suggests that postdiagnosis physical activity might restrict available energy, thereby inhibiting the growth of CDKN1B-expressing tumors. Second, postdiagnosis physical activity might lead to a beneficial effect that reduces PTGS2 (COX2). PTGS2 is a crucial inflammatory response and is related to colorectal carcinogenesis. Yamauchi and colleagues[49] reported that physically active patients with PTCG2-expressing tumors had better survival than physically active patients without a PTCG2-expressing tumor. Finally, WNT-CTNNB1 signaling could be a key regulator of energy metabolism and carcinogenesis. When patients with colon cancer had a negative status for nuclear CTNNB1, postdiagnosis physical activity was found to have a favorable association with colorectal cancer–specific survival.[31] Further studies are required to find other related molecular mechanisms.

Table 5
Prospective cohort studies of postdiagnosis physical activity and survival outcomes in patients with colorectal cancer

Authors, Ref. Year, Name of Cohort, Country	Study Participants	Median Years of Follow-Up	Relative Risk/Hazard Ratio (95% Confidence Interval)		Adjustment Factors
Meyerhardt et al,[15] 2006, Nurses' Health Study, USA	554 Female Colon and rectal	9.6	**CRC-specific mortality**		Age of diagnosis, stage, tumor differentiation, year of diagnosis, time between study entry to questionnaire, BMI, smoking, receipt of chemotherapy, time from diagnosis to physical activity measurement
			<3 MET-h/wk	Referent	
			3–8.9	0.92 (0.50–1.69)	
			9–17.9	0.57 (0.27–1.20)	
			≥18	0.39 (0.18–0.82)	
			All-cause mortality		
			<3 MET-h/wk	Referent	
			3–8.9	0.77 (0.48–1.23)	
			9–17.9	0.50 (0.28–0.90)	
			≥18	0.43 (0.25–0.74)	
Meyerhardt et al,[43] 2006, CALGB 89803, USA	832 both genders Colon	3.8	**Disease-free survival**		Sex, age, depth of invasion through bowel wall, number of positive lymph node, presence of clinical perforation at time of surgery, presence of bowel obstruction, baseline carcinoembryonic antigen, grade of tumor differentiation, baseline performance status, treatment arm, weight change between first and second questionnaire, BMI at the time of second questionnaire, and time between study entry and completion of second questionnaire
			<3 MET-h/wk	Referent	
			3–8.9	0.87 (0.58–1.29)	
			9–17	0.90 (0.57–1.40)	
			18–26.9	0.51 (0.26–0.97)	
			≥27	0.55 (0.33–0.91)	
			Recurrence-free survival		
			<3 MET-h/wk	Referent	
			3–8.9	0.86 (0.57–1.30)	
			9–17	0.89 (0.55–1.42)	
			18–26.9	0.51 (0.26–1.01)	
			≥27	0.60 (0.36–1.01)	
			All-cause mortality		
			<3 MET-h/wk	Referent	
			3–8.9	0.85 (0.49–1.49)	
			9–17	0.71 (0.36–1.41)	
			18–26.9	0.71 (0.32–1.59)	
			≥27	0.37 (0.16–0.82)	

Meyerhardt et al,[16] 2009, Health Professionals Follow-Up Study, USA	661 Male Colon and rectal	8.6	**CRC-specific mortality**		Age, stage, year of diagnosis, disease stage, tumor differentiation, tumor location, BMI, smoking
			<3 MET-h/wk	*Referent*	
			3.1–9	1.06 (0.55–2.08)	
			9.1–18	1.30 (0.65–2.59)	
			18.1–27	0.76 (0.33–1.77)	
			≥27	0.47 (0.24–0.92)	
			All-cause mortality		
			<3 MET-h/wk	*Referent*	
			3.1–9	1.00 (0.68–1.48)	
			9.1–18	1.12 (0.74–1.70)	
			18.1–27	0.74 (0.46–1.20)	
			≥27	0.59 (0.41–0.86)	
Baade et al,[5] 2011, Queensland, Australia	1825 both genders Colon and rectal	4.9	**CRC-specific mortality**		Age, sex, stage at diagnosis, smoking, site of tumor, treatment (surgery only vs surgery and adjuvant therapy)
			Sedentary	*Referent*	
			Insufficiently active	0.90 (0.69–1.17)	
			Sufficiently active	0.88 (0.68–1.15)	
			All-cause mortality		
			Sedentary	*Referent*	
			Insufficiently active	0.72 (0.57–0.90)	
			Sufficiently active	0.75 (0.60–0.94)	

(continued on next page)

Table 5
(continued)

Authors,[Ref.] Year, Name of Cohort, Country	Study Participants	Median Years of Follow-Up	Relative Risk/Hazard Ratio (95% Confidence Interval)		Adjustment Factors
Kuiper et al,[12] 2012, Women's Health Initiative, USA	676 Female Colon and rectal	11.9	**CRC-specific mortality**		Age, study arm, time from diagnosis to measurement, prediagnostic BMI, tumor stage, ethnicity, education, alcohol, smoking, hormone therapy use
			0 MET-h/wk	*Referent*	
			>0–2.9	0.49 (0.21–1.14)	
			3.0–8.9	0.30 (0.12–0.73)	
			9.0–17.9	0.53 (0.22–1.25)	
			≥27	0.29 (0.11–0.77)	
			All-cause mortality		
			0 MET-h/wk	*Referent*	
			>0–2.9	0.71 (0.40–1.30)	
			3.0–8.9	0.42 (0.23–0.77)	
			9.0–17.9	0.57 (0.31–1.07)	
			≥27	0.41 (0.21–0.81)	
Campbell et al,[17] 2013, Cancer Prevention Study-II, USA	1800 both genders Colon and rectal	6.8	**CRC-specific mortality**		Age, sex, smoking status, BMI, red meat intake, tumor stage, leisure time spent sitting, education
			<3.5 MET-h/wk	*Referent*	
			3.5–<8.75	1.00 (0.64–1.56)	
			≥8.75	0.87 (0.61–1.24)	
			All-cause mortality		
			<3.5 MET-h/wk	*Referent*	
			3.5–<8.75	0.78 (0.60–1.00)	
			≥8.75	0.58 (0.47–0.71)	

Abbreviation: MET-h/wk, metabolic-equivalent task hours per week.

Table 6
Prospective cohort studies of postdiagnosis diet and survival outcomes in patients with colorectal cancer

Authors,[Ref.] Year, Name of Cohort, Country	Study Participants	Median Years of Follow-Up	Dietary Measure	Relative Risk/Hazard Ratio (95% Confidence Interval)	Adjustment Factors
Meyerhardt et al,[9] 2007, National Cancer Institute-sponsored Cancer and Leukemia Group B (CALGB) 89,803, USA	1009 both genders Colon	5.3	Western pattern diet	**Disease-free survival** Highest vs lowest quintile 3.25 (2.04–5.19) **Recurrence-free survival** Highest vs lowest quintile 2.85 (1.75–4.63) **Overall survival** Highest vs lowest quintile 2.32 (1.36–3.96)	Stage, age, nodal stage, BMI, physical activity, baseline performance status, or treatment group
Meyerhardt et al,[44] 2012, National Cancer Institute-sponsored Cancer and Leukemia Group B (CALGB) 89,803, USA	1011 both genders Colon	7.3	Glycemic load	**Disease-free survival** Highest vs lowest quintile 1.79 (1.29–2.48) **Recurrence-free survival** Highest vs lowest quintile 1.98 (1.39–2.80) **Overall survival** Highest vs lowest quintile 1.76 (1.22–2.54)	Sex, age, depth of invasion through bowel wall, number of positive lymph nodes, baseline performance status, treatment group, body mass index, physical activity level, and cereal fiber intake
McCullough et al,[8] 2013, Cancer Prevention Study-II Nutrition Cohort, USA	1186 both genders Colon and rectal	7.6	Red and processed meat	**CRC-specific mortality** Highest vs lowest quartile 1.34 (0.77–2.33) **Overall mortality** Highest vs lowest quintile 1.09 (0.81–1.48)	Age at diagnosis, sex, tumor stage at diagnosis, energy intake. weight change

ENERGY BALANCE INTERVENTION STUDIES IN SURVIVORS OF COLORECTAL CANCER

All reported intervention studies to date in survivors of colorectal cancer have examined quality-of-life–related end points.[50–52] At present there is one ongoing intervention study to specifically study disease-free survival in survivors of stage II and III colorectal cancer.[50] Courneya and colleagues[50] continue to study the effect of physical activity intervention over a 3-year period, and how that intervention affected recurrences, mortality, physical functioning, quality of life, and biological correlative markers for patients with colon cancer. The study is sponsored by the National Cancer Institute of Canada and has ongoing accrual in Canada and Australia. Additional research opportunities exist that need to address other approaches to extending the mortality of colorectal cancer, which include developing diverse tailored intervention programs, such as home-based and Web-based programs that change the patient's modifiable lifestyle factors.

SUMMARY

Lifestyle factors that include obesity, physical activity, and diet are emerging as potential critical elements in improving survival outcomes for colorectal cancer. The evidence for an association between colorectal cancer mortality and modifiable lifestyle factors is growing. Changes in individual health behaviors both before and after a diagnosis of colorectal cancer may improve outcomes of survivors. Several studies have indicated that maintaining a normal weight, participating in regular physical activity, and eating a healthy diet may be important preventive steps that leading to improved survival outcomes. Moreover, several epigenetic studies have demonstrated, at the cellular level, the possible mechanisms of colorectal cancer that can be positively influenced by changing one's lifestyle. However, extended lifestyle intervention studies, along with additional randomized trials and epigenetic studies, are needed to provide firm evidence about the effect of lifestyle factors (including obesity, physical activity, and diet) on survival outcomes of colorectal cancer.

REFERENCES

1. American Cancer Society. Colorectal cancer facts & figures. Atlanta (GA): American Cancer Society; 2011.
2. Ferlay J, Parkin DM, Steliarova-Foucher E. Estimates of cancer incidence and mortality in Europe in 2008. Eur J Cancer 2010;46:765–81.
3. Chan AT, Giovannucci EL. Primary prevention of colorectal cancer. Gastroenterology 2010;138:2029–43.e10.
4. Ligibel J. Lifestyle factors in cancer survivorship. J Clin Oncol 2012;30:3697–704.
5. Baade PD, Meng X, Youl PH, et al. The impact of body mass index and physical activity on mortality among patients with colorectal cancer in Queensland, Australia. Cancer Epidemiol Biomarkers Prev 2011;20:1410–20.
6. Campbell PT, Newton CC, Dehal AN, et al. Impact of body mass index on survival after colorectal cancer diagnosis: the Cancer Prevention Study-II Nutrition Cohort. J Clin Oncol 2012;30:42–52.
7. Je Y, Jeon JY, Giovannucci EL, et al. Association between physical activity and mortality in colorectal cancer: a meta-analysis of prospective cohort studies. Int J Cancer 2013;133:1905–13.
8. McCullough ML, Gapstur SM, Shah R, et al. Association between red and processed meat intake and mortality among colorectal cancer survivors. J Clin Oncol 2013;31:2773–82.

9. Meyerhardt JA, Niedzwiecki D, Hollis D, et al. Association of dietary patterns with cancer recurrence and survival in patients with stage III colon cancer. JAMA 2007;298:754–64.

10. Doria-Rose VP, Newcomb PA, Morimoto LM, et al. Body mass index and the risk of death following the diagnosis of colorectal cancer in postmenopausal women (United States). Cancer Causes Control 2006;17:63–70.

11. Prizment AE, Flood A, Anderson KE, et al. Survival of women with colon cancer in relation to precancer anthropometric characteristics: the Iowa Women's Health Study. Cancer Epidemiol Biomarkers Prev 2010;19:2229–37.

12. Kuiper JG, Phipps AI, Neuhouser ML, et al. Recreational physical activity, body mass index, and survival in women with colorectal cancer. Cancer Causes Control 2012;23:1939–48.

13. Pelser C, Arem H, Pfeiffer RM, et al. Prediagnostic lifestyle factors and survival after colon and rectal cancer diagnosis in the National Institutes of Health (NIH)-AARP Diet and Health Study. Cancer 2014;120(10):1540–7.

14. Haydon AM, Macinnis RJ, English DR, et al. Effect of physical activity and body size on survival after diagnosis with colorectal cancer. Gut 2006;55:62–7.

15. Meyerhardt JA, Giovannucci EL, Holmes MD, et al. Physical activity and survival after colorectal cancer diagnosis. J Clin Oncol 2006;24:3527–34.

16. Meyerhardt JA, Ogino S, Kirkner GJ, et al. Interaction of molecular markers and physical activity on mortality in patients with colon cancer. Clin Cancer Res 2009; 15:5931–6.

17. Campbell PT, Patel AV, Newton CC, et al. Associations of recreational physical activity and leisure time spent sitting with colorectal cancer survival. J Clin Oncol 2013;31:876–85.

18. Giovannucci E. Modifiable risk factors for colon cancer. Gastroenterol Clin North Am 2002;31:925–43.

19. Zell JA, Ignatenko NA, Yerushalmi HF, et al. Risk and risk reduction involving arginine intake and meat consumption in colorectal tumorigenesis and survival. Int J Cancer 2007;120:459–68.

20. Zhu Y, Wu H, Wang PP, et al. Dietary patterns and colorectal cancer recurrence and survival: a cohort study. BMJ Open 2013;7;3(2).

21. Chan DS, Lau R, Aune D, et al. Red and processed meat and colorectal cancer incidence: meta-analysis of prospective studies. PLoS One 2011;6:e20456.

22. Giovannucci E. Insulin, insulin-like growth factors and colon cancer: a review of the evidence. J Nutr 2001;131:3109S–20S.

23. Wolpin BM, Meyerhardt JA, Chan AT, et al. Insulin, the insulin-like growth factor axis, and mortality in patients with nonmetastatic colorectal cancer. J Clin Oncol 2009;27:176–85.

24. Aparicio T, Kotelevets L, Tsocas A, et al. Leptin stimulates the proliferation of human colon cancer cells in vitro but does not promote the growth of colon cancer xenografts in nude mice or intestinal tumorigenesis in Apc(Min/+) mice. Gut 2005;54:1136–45.

25. Ogunwobi OO, Beales IL. The anti-apoptotic and growth stimulatory actions of leptin in human colon cancer cells involves activation of JNK mitogen activated protein kinase, JAK2 and PI3 kinase/Akt. Int J Colorectal Dis 2007;22: 401–9.

26. Zins K, Abraham D, Sioud M, et al. Colon cancer cell-derived tumor necrosis factor-alpha mediates the tumor growth-promoting response in macrophages by up-regulating the colony-stimulating factor-1 pathway. Cancer Res 2007;67: 1038–45.

27. Street ME, Miraki-Moud F, Sanderson IR, et al. Interleukin-1beta (IL-1beta) and IL-6 modulate insulin-like growth factor-binding protein (IGFBP) secretion in colon cancer epithelial (Caco-2) cells. J Endocrinol 2003;179:405–15.

28. Power ML, Schulkin J. Sex differences in fat storage, fat metabolism, and the health risks from obesity: possible evolutionary origins. Br J Nutr 2008;99:931–40.

29. Chung YW, Han DS, Park YK, et al. Association of obesity, serum glucose and lipids with the risk of advanced colorectal adenoma and cancer: a case-control study in Korea. Dig Liver Dis 2006;38:668–72.

30. Morikawa T, Kuchiba A, Lochhead P, et al. Prospective analysis of body mass index, physical activity, and colorectal cancer risk associated with beta-catenin (CTNNB1) status. Cancer Res 2013;73:1600–10.

31. Morikawa T, Kuchiba A, Yamauchi M, et al. Association of CTNNB1 (beta-catenin) alterations, body mass index, and physical activity with survival in patients with colorectal cancer. JAMA 2011;305:1685–94.

32. Sugimura T. Carcinogenicity of mutagenic heterocyclic amines formed during the cooking process. Mutat Res 1985;150:33–41.

33. O'Callaghan NJ, Toden S, Bird AR, et al. Colonocyte telomere shortening is greater with dietary red meat than white meat and is attenuated by resistant starch. Clin Nutr 2012;31:60–4.

34. Bastide NM, Pierre FH, Corpet DE. Heme iron from meat and risk of colorectal cancer: a meta-analysis and a review of the mechanisms involved. Cancer Prev Res (Phila) 2011;4:177–84.

35. Cross AJ, Sinha R. Meat-related mutagens/carcinogens in the etiology of colorectal cancer. Environ Mol Mutagen 2004;44:44–55.

36. Meyerhardt JA, Catalano PJ, Haller DG, et al. Influence of body mass index on outcomes and treatment-related toxicity in patients with colon carcinoma. Cancer 2003;98:484–95.

37. Dignam JJ, Polite BN, Yothers G, et al. Body mass index and outcomes in patients who receive adjuvant chemotherapy for colon cancer. J Natl Cancer Inst 2006;98:1647–54.

38. Meyerhardt JA, Niedzwiecki D, Hollis D, et al. Impact of body mass index and weight change after treatment on cancer recurrence and survival in patients with stage III colon cancer: findings from Cancer and Leukemia Group B 89803. J Clin Oncol 2008;26:4109–15.

39. Sinicrope FA, Foster NR, Sargent DJ, et al. Obesity is an independent prognostic variable in colon cancer survivors. Clin Cancer Res 2010;16:1884–93.

40. Chin CC, Kuo YH, Yeh CY, et al. Role of body mass index in colon cancer patients in Taiwan. World J Gastroenterol 2012;18:4191–8.

41. Sinicrope FA, Foster NR, Yothers G, et al. Body mass index at diagnosis and survival among colon cancer patients enrolled in clinical trials of adjuvant chemotherapy. Cancer 2013;119:1528–36.

42. Jeon JY, Meyerhardt JA. Energy in and energy out: what matters for survivors of colorectal cancer? J Clin Oncol 2012;30:7–10.

43. Meyerhardt JA, Heseltine D, Niedzwiecki D, et al. Impact of physical activity on cancer recurrence and survival in patients with stage III colon cancer: findings from CALGB 89803. J Clin Oncol 2006;24:3535–41.

44. Meyerhardt JA, Sato K, Niedzwiecki D, et al. Dietary glycemic load and cancer recurrence and survival in patients with stage III colon cancer: findings from CALGB 89803. J Natl Cancer Inst 2012;104:1702–11.

45. Hiromura K, Monkawa T, Petermann AT, et al. Insulin is a potent survival factor in mesangial cells: role of the PI3-kinase/Akt pathway. Kidney Int 2002;61:1312–21.

46. Cantrell LA, Zhou C, Mendivil A, et al. Metformin is a potent inhibitor of endometrial cancer cell proliferation–implications for a novel treatment strategy. Gynecol Oncol 2010;116:92–8.

47. Lee DH, Kim JY, Lee MK, et al. Effects of a 12-week home-based exercise program on the level of physical activity, insulin, and cytokines in colorectal cancer survivors: a pilot study. Support Care Cancer 2013;21:2537–45.

48. Ogino S, Nosho K, Meyerhardt JA, et al. Cohort study of fatty acid synthase expression and patient survival in colon cancer. J Clin Oncol 2008;26:5713–20.

49. Yamauchi M, Lochhead P, Imamura Y, et al. Physical activity, tumor PTGS2 expression, and survival in patients with colorectal cancer. Cancer Epidemiol Biomarkers Prev 2013;22:1142–52.

50. Courneya KS, Booth CM, Gill S, et al. The Colon Health and Life-Long Exercise Change trial: a randomized trial of the National Cancer Institute of Canada Clinical Trials Group. Curr Oncol 2008;15:279–85.

51. Ligibel JA, Meyerhardt J, Pierce JP, et al. Impact of a telephone-based physical activity intervention upon exercise behaviors and fitness in cancer survivors enrolled in a cooperative group setting. Breast Cancer Res Treat 2012;132: 205–13.

52. Pinto BM, Papandonatos GD, Goldstein MG, et al. Home-based physical activity intervention for colorectal cancer survivors. Psychooncology 2013;22:54–64.

53. Meyerhardt JA, Tepper JE, Niedzwiecki D, et al. Impact of body mass index on outcomes and treatment-related toxicity in patients with stage II and III rectal cancer: findings from Intergroup Trial 0114. J Clin Oncol 2004;22:648–57.

Diagnosis and Management of DNA Mismatch Repair-Deficient Colorectal Cancer

Zsofia K. Stadler, MD

KEYWORDS

• Microsatellite instability • Mismatch repair deficiency • Colorectal cancer prognosis

KEY POINTS

• Defective DNA mismatch repair (MMR-D), also referred to as microsatellite instability (MSI-H), is present in approximately 15% of colorectal cancers (CRCs).

• In most cases, MMR-D/MSI-H in colorectal tumors is caused by a noninherited epigenetic event; however, in about one-third of cases, it is caused by Lynch syndrome.

• Identification of MMR-D/MSI-H in patients with CRC may lead to a diagnosis of Lynch syndrome, with important clinical implications for future cancer surveillance and risk-reduction options for the patient as well as for at-risk family members.

• MMR-D/MSI-H is associated with distinct clinical and pathologic features, including right-sided colon predominance, early stage at diagnosis, prominent lymphocytic infiltrate, and a poorly differentiated mucinous adenocarcinoma, often showing a medullary component.

• Although MMR-D/MSI-H in CRC is associated with a favorable prognosis, it also seems to predict for a lack of benefit from 5-fluorouracil chemotherapy.

INTRODUCTION

Colorectal cancers (CRCs) may be divided via molecular phenotyping into tumors with normal DNA mismatch repair (MMR) function and those with DNA MMR deficiency (MMR-D), representing ~15% of CRCs.[1,2] The hallmark of MMR-D CRC is a distinct type of genomic instability, referred to as high-frequency microsatellite instability (MSI-H).[3] MMR-D/MSI-H is associated with specific clinical and pathologic features, and in some cases, may provide the initial clinical indication suggesting the presence of Lynch syndrome, an inherited form of CRC, characterized by germline genetic defects in one of the DNA MMR genes (*MLH1, MSH2, MSH6, PMS2, EPCAM*). Lynch

Clinical Genetics Service, Department of Medicine, Memorial Sloan Kettering Cancer Center, 1275 York Avenue, New York, NY 10065, USA
E-mail address: stadlerz@mskcc.org

Hematol Oncol Clin N Am 29 (2015) 29–41
http://dx.doi.org/10.1016/j.hoc.2014.09.008
0889-8588/15/$ – see front matter © 2015 Elsevier Inc. All rights reserved.

syndrome remains significantly underdiagnosed, and recent measures to expand screening of patients with Lynch-associated cancers, including those with CRC and endometrial cancer, provides one of the most effective ways to identify at-risk families.[4,5] The MMR-D/MSI-H phenotype also serves as an important prognostic and predictive marker in CRC. Although MMR-D/MSI-H CRCs tend to be early stage at diagnosis and are associated with a good prognosis, the value of 5-fluorouracil (5-FU) as an effective chemotherapeutic treatment of this type of CRC has been debated. As our understanding of MMR-D/MSI-H CRCs continues to evolve, oncologists remain at the forefront of diagnosing, treating, and managing patients with this unique subtype of CRC and ensuring that, for appropriate patients, referral to clinical cancer genetics for Lynch syndrome evaluation is implemented.

THE ADENOMA-CARCINOMA MODEL OF COLORECTAL CANCER

The development of CRCs via the adenoma-carcinoma sequence, initially described by Fearon and Vogelstein in 1990,[6] proposed a multistep genetic model of CRC carcinogenesis. Most CRCs arise along the chromosomal instability pathway, characterized by widespread imbalances in chromosome number (aneuploidy) and loss of heterozygosity, as well as the accumulation of characteristic mutations in tumor suppressor genes and oncogenes critical for CRC initiation and progression.[7,8] The second pathway, accounting for 15% to 20% of CRCs, results from defective DNA MMR, which leads to the molecular phenomenon of MSI-H shown within the tumor.[3,9] Microsatellites are short, tandemly repeated DNA sequences that are distributed throughout the human genome and consist of mononucleotide, dinucleotide, or higher-order DNA base repeats.[1] Such repetitive sequences are prone to the accumulation of mutations mostly because of base-base mismatches and insertion-deletion loops. The correction of errors in microsatellites is performed by the MMR proteins, the most notable of which are MLH1, MSH2, MSH6, and PMS2. In tumors with MMR-D, either because of germline, somatic, or epigenetic inactivation, the correction of such mutations is impaired, leading to the accumulation of DNA errors, resulting in the MSI-H phenotype.

In most cases, MMR-D is a result of an epigenetic phenomenon in the tumor, most commonly hypermethylation of the *MLH1* promoter, which leads to the development of a sporadic (noninherited) CRC.[10,11] However, in about 30% of cases, MMR-D is secondary to a germline mutation in one of the MMR genes, leading to a diagnosis of Lynch syndrome, an inherited form of CRC. Deciphering the cause of the MMR-D is of upmost importance, because it helps to differentiate sporadic from inherited forms of colon cancer.

SCREENING FOR DEFECTIVE DNA MISMATCH REPAIR/HIGH-FREQUENCY MICROSATELLITE INSTABILITY IN PATIENTS WITH COLORECTAL CANCER: SHOULD A UNIVERSAL APPROACH BE APPLIED?

The identification of the MMR-D/MSI-H phenotype in a colorectal tumor may be the first indication that a patient may have a diagnosis of Lynch syndrome. Patients identified to have Lynch syndrome benefit from life-saving cancer surveillance measures.[12] In addition, their at-risk family members would benefit from predictive genetic testing and, if needed, implementation of high-risk cancer surveillance. Although measures aimed at increasing awareness about hereditary CRC, both among individuals as well as among physicians, may be undertaken, one of the most effective ways to identify potential at-risk Lynch families is by evaluating patients who are diagnosed with either CRC or endometrial cancer, the 2 most common Lynch-associated malignancies.

Originally, the Amsterdam criteria and subsequently, the Revised Bethesda guidelines, have served as criteria to select patients with CRC or endometrial cancer in whom further evaluation for MMR-D/MSI-H was indicated.[13,14] However, in the clinical setting these criteria have proved to be cumbersome to implement and lack specificity and sensitivity. Some groups have recommended expansion of the criteria for MMR/MSI testing to either universal testing, with testing of all patients with CRC, or to include all individuals with CRC diagnosed younger than 70 years. Using universal testing, Lynch syndrome was diagnosed in 2.4% to 3.7% of all unselected patients with CRC.[4,15,16] Implementing universal screening for endometrial cancer yielded similar results, with about 1.8% to 3.9% of patients being diagnosed with Lynch syndrome.[5,17] In the CRC cases, a Lynch syndrome diagnosis would have been missed in ~12% to 28% of patients if the Revised Bethesda guidelines were used for selection criteria.[4,15,16] More expansive testing of CRC and endometrial cases has also proved to be cost effective.[18,19]

Based on these data, the Mallorca group, consisting of European experts in Lynch syndrome, the Evaluation of Genomic Applications in Practice and Prevention Working Group, and the National Comprehensive Cancer Network have recently updated their recommendations to suggest that either all patients with CRC or all patients with CRC younger than 70 years at diagnosis, and those 70 years or older who meet Bethesda guidelines, should undergo testing by either immunohistochemistry (IHC) or MSI for Lynch syndrome.[20–22] Implementation of such reflex testing is already occurring across large medical centers, with a recent study[23] suggesting that the specific implementation procedures influenced patient follow-through with genetic testing after an initial positive screening test. For example, institutions with a high level of involvement of genetic counselors in the tracking and communicating of screening results improved patient follow-through and reduced barriers to patient contact.[23]

IDENTIFICATION OF DEFECTIVE DNA MISMATCH REPAIR/HIGH-FREQUENCY MICROSATELLITE INSTABILITY TUMORS

Two accepted methods for the detection of MMR-D are available. MSI testing relies on polymerase chain reaction for amplification of specific microsatellites repeats. The original accepted panel of 5 microsatellite markers, referred to as the Bethesda panel, includes 2 mononucleotides (BAT-25, BAT-26) and 3 dinucleotides (D5S346, D2S123, D17S250).[24,25] The presence of instability is determined based on comparison of the length of a specific microsatellite marker in the tumor versus the normal DNA, such as adjacent colonic mucosa or a blood sample. Instability in 2 or more markers is defined as an MSI-high tumor, whereas those with 1 unstable marker are designated MSI low.[26] For a sample to be microsatellite stable (MSS), no instability in any of the markers should be present. Given concerns over limited sensitivity of dinucleotide repeats, the 2002 National Cancer Institute workshop made further revisions, with recommendations to include a secondary panel of mononucleotide markers, such as BAT-40, to exclude MSI-low cases in which only a dinucleotide repeat is mutated.[14,26]

In 1996, monoclonal antibodies against MMR proteins became available, rendering IHC detection of MMR proteins possible.[27] A lack of expression of 1 or more of these proteins is diagnostic of MMR-D, with the specific pattern of expression also helping to pinpoint which gene is most likely to harbor a mutation or may be inactivated by another mechanism (**Table 1**).[27] Initial concerns over lower sensitivity of IHC as opposed to MSI screening have largely been overcome with the introduction of the

Table 1
Commonly observed patterns of DNA MMR protein expression by IHC staining

Protein Expression by IHC Staining					
MLH1	MSH2	MSH6	PMS2	MMR Status	Most Likely Inactivated Gene
Present	Present	Present	Present	Proficient	None
Absent	Present	Present	Absent	Deficient	*MLH1* (epigenetic or germline)
Present	Present	Present	Absent	Deficient	*PMS2*
Present	Absent	Absent	Present	Deficient	*MSH2*, possibly *EPCAM*
Present	Present	Absent	Present	Deficient	*MSH6*

4-antibody panel (MLH1, MSH2, MSH6, PMS2). In the clinical setting, both IHC and MSI testing are used broadly and are essentially interchangeable techniques with greater than 90% concordance and similar sensitivity of around 85% to 92%.[27] At our institution, the preference to use IHC as opposed to MSI testing for initial screening was largely based on the ability of IHC to pinpoint which genes should be targeted for subsequent germline analysis in MMR-D cases, thereby simplifying the genetic testing process.

DEFECTIVE DNA MISMATCH REPAIR/HIGH-FREQUENCY MICROSATELLITE INSTABILITY COLORECTAL CANCER: MAKING THE DIAGNOSIS OF LYNCH SYNDROME

An MSI-H or an abnormal IHC result does not distinguish between a somatic (sporadic) versus a germline (inherited) defect in the MMR system. Without further analysis, the cause of the defect remains elusive. In approximately two-thirds of cases, MSI-H indicates a sporadic CRC, with the molecular phenomenon being caused by an epigenetic event, most commonly *MLH1* promoter hypermethylation, leading to *MLH1* gene inactivation. In about 70% of such promoter hypermethylated MSI-H cases, the presence of a *BRAF* V600E mutation can be identified.[28] The presence of a *BRAF* V600E mutation in a colorectal tumor would make the diagnosis of Lynch syndrome less likely, and together with an absence of suggestive family history, may reassure clinicians of the sporadic cause of the MSI-H CRC.[29,30] Cases of *BRAF* mutated tumors in Lynch syndrome–associated CRCs have been reported, and therefore a careful review of the clinical and family history should be undertaken to determine whether further genetic counseling/testing is indicated.[30] In many centers, an MSI-H CRC or a CRC showing loss of MLH1/PMS2 protein expression is immediately tested via direct *MLH1* hypermethylation analysis or *BRAF* V600E mutation analysis. These are generally not considered genetic tests but are used for risk stratification to determine which patients may benefit from subsequent genetic testing.

In one-third of MSI-H tumors, the molecular defect is secondary to a germline mutation in one of the MMR genes, diagnostic of Lynch syndrome. In patients with CRC in whom Lynch syndrome is suspected based on early age at diagnosis or family history of Lynch-associated malignancies, an abnormal IHC or MSI-H result should prompt referral for genetic counseling and genetic testing. If IHC was performed, then the specific protein expression loss helps guide genetic testing (see **Table 1**). For example, in a tumor with absence of MSH2 and MSH6 expression, genetic testing for mutations in the MSH2 gene should be undertaken initially. Identification of a genetic mutation confirms the diagnosis of Lynch syndrome. In such patients, appropriate cancer surveillance and options for cancer risk reduction need to be reviewed and implemented.

Moreover, expansion of genetic counseling and testing for family members should be undertaken.

A difficult clinical situation that arises not infrequently is that workup of a patient with an MSI-H or MMR-D CRC results in ambiguous or uninformative results with respect to the origin of the MMR defect. For example, in a young patient with CRC with absence of MLH1/PMS2 protein expression, genetic testing of the *MLH1* and *PMS2* genes may be unrevealing, with no mutation identified. Coupled with the absence of MLH1 promoter hypermethylation and absence of a BRAF mutation, in such a clinical circumstance, Lynch syndrome cannot be ruled out. In such situations, a careful evaluation of the family history may help to identify other cancer-affected family members whose tumors could be evaluated for the MMR-D/MSI-H molecular signature and, if positive, would confirm the presence of an occult mutation. These cases require the careful input of genetic counselors and cancer geneticists for recommendations for appropriate cancer surveillance for both the patient and at-risk family members.

CLINICAL AND PATHOLOGIC FEATURES OF DEFECTIVE DNA MISMATCH REPAIR/HIGH-FREQUENCY MICROSATELLITE INSTABILITY COLORECTAL CANCERS

Regardless of the cause of the MMR deficiency, MMR-D/MSI-H CRCs seem to be associated with distinct clinical and pathologic features, which often serve as the initial clue that a particular tumor may harbor an MMR defect (**Table 2**). As opposed to the 25% of MSS colorectal tumors, 85% of MMR-D/MSI-H tumors are proximal to the splenic flexure. Moreover, the age distribution of MMR-D/MSI-H tumors seems to be bimodal, with about 24% of patients with CRC younger than 40 years and 19% older than 70 years having MSI-H tumors, as opposed to only 8% of patients with CRC aged between 50 and 59 years.[31] This U-shaped age distribution reflects the higher prevalence of Lynch-associated MMR-D/MSI-H CRCs in young patients and the similarly higher prevalence of sporadic MMR-D/MSI-H phenotype observed in older patients.

Despite the improved prognosis (see later discussion) associated with the MMR-D/MSI-H phenotype, such tumors tend to show a higher histologic grade and are often mucinous tumors with presence of signet-ring cells. A recently recognized feature is

Table 2
Clinical and pathologic features of MMR-D/MSI-H CRCs

Right-colon predominance
Mucinous, signet-ring cells
Tumor-infiltrating lymphocytes, Crohn-like nodular infiltrate
Absence of necrotic cellular debris
Poorly differentiated adenocarcinoma (medullary subtype)
Low pathologic stage

Sporadic, Noninherited MMR-D	Inherited MMR-D (Lynch Syndrome)
Presence of epigenetic *MLH1* promoter hypermethylation	Presence of a germline mutation in one of the MMR genes (*MLH1, MSH2, MSH6, PMS2*)
Often positive for *V600E* BRAF somatic mutation	Generally, no somatic BRAF mutation identified
More common in older and female patients	Increased risk of synchronous and metachronous CRC Risk of extracolonic cancers (eg, endometrial, ovarian, gastric, ureter, pancreas) Requires genetic counseling and testing of at-risk family members

the presence of the distinct medullary subtype of colorectal adenocarcinoma, associated with a unique histologic appearance and a more favorable prognosis compared with standard poorly differentiated colonic carcinomas. Medullary carcinomas are generally associated with a right-sided predominance, older female patients, and a lower incidence of lymph node metastases. Morphologic features of such tumors are characterized by a syncytial growth pattern and large vesicular nuclei, with conspicuous nucleoli and prominent peritumoral lymphocytic infiltrates. Because there is significant morphologic overlap between medullary carcinomas and poorly differentiated carcinomas, these may be difficult to differentiate. However, the presence of medullary carcinoma subtype, even if categorized under a poorly differentiated carcinoma, is associated with a favorable prognosis. In 1 study, MLH1 antibody staining was absent in nearly 80% of medullary carcinomas, indicating the close association of MMR-D/MSI-H with this subtype of CRC. Other common features include prominent tumor-infiltrating lymphocytes, lack of necrotic debris, and a Crohn-like lymphocytic host reaction. These distinct histologic features evoke the possible presence of MMR-D/MSI-H, prompting the pathologist to perform subsequent MSI or IHC testing.

DEFECTIVE DNA MISMATCH REPAIR/HIGH-FREQUENCY MICROSATELLITE INSTABILITY AS A PROGNOSTIC MARKER IN COLORECTAL CANCER

In addition to the distinct clinicopathologic features, numerous studies have also suggested a favorable prognosis of MMR-D/MSI-H colon tumors. Patients with MMR-D/MSI-H tumors tend to have a lower tumor stage at diagnosis and rarely develop metastatic disease. When assessed stage by stage, the presence of MMR-D/MSI-H is noted in ~20% of stage I/II, ~12% of stage III, but only ~4% of stage IV patients, again suggesting an association with earlier stage of disease. Substantial evidence has accumulated from retrospective studies, population-based studies, as well as a meta-analysis[32] to suggest a more favorable prognosis in MMR-D/MSI-H colorectal tumors.

In 2000, Gryfe and colleagues[33] initially reported an association of MSI-H status, with a survival advantage that was independent of all standard prognostic features. This analysis was limited to CRCs diagnosed at age 50 years or younger, limiting the generalizability of this result to all patients with CRC. In the seminal 2003 publication by Ribic and colleagues,[34] of patients with stage II and III colon cancer who did not receive adjuvant chemotherapy, those with MMR-D/MSI-H had significantly improved overall survival compared with MMR-P/MSS tumors with a hazard ratio (HR) for death of 0.31 (95% confidence interval [CI], 0.14–0.72, $P = .004$).The improved prognosis associated with MMR-D/MSI-H was despite the presence of a higher percentage of poorly differentiated tumors in the MMR-D/MSI-H group (26% vs 9%).[34] A subsequent meta-analyses of 32 studies,[32] including a total of 7642 patients with CRC, including all stages of disease, also found a favorable overall survival in the 1277 MSI-H tumors with an HR of 0.65 (95% CI, 0.59–0.71). When the analysis was restricted to clinical trials only, the benefit was maintained with an HR of 0.69. In this meta-analysis, both treated (5-FU–based adjuvant treatment) and untreated patients were included from phase 3 randomized trials.[32] In the Quick And Simple And Reliable (QUASAR) trial assessing stage II CRCs, MMR-D was an independent prognostic factor, with an improvement in survival with an HR of 0.31. Nonetheless, several studies do not corroborate the survival advantage associated with MMR-D/MSI-H tumors.[35,36] Such discrepant results may be caused by limited power to detect prognostic differences because of small sample size, different methodologies used for the assessment of defective MMR (ie, 4 vs 2 antibody IHC testing;

MSI analysis with different panel and numbers of markers), different treatment and stage of disease included in the analysis, and selection bias. Because patients with MMR-D/MSI-H caused by Lynch syndrome comprise an even smaller group (~2–3% of all CRCs), power to detect prognostic differences specifically for patients with Lynch syndrome is even more limited. Nonetheless, based on the preponderance of evidence, it is generally well accepted that MMR-D/MSI-H tumors are associated with an improved prognosis, with the more contentious issue being the importance of MMR-D/MSI-H status as a predictive marker in the treatment of CRC.

DEFECTIVE DNA MISMATCH REPAIR/HIGH-FREQUENCY MICROSATELLITE INSTABILITY STATUS AS A PREDICTIVE MARKER IN COLORECTAL CANCER
5-Fluorouracil–Based Chemotherapy

In addition to being a prognostic marker for CRC outcome, the MMR-D/MSI-H phenotype has also been implicated as a predictive marker, with studies suggesting that such tumors do not derive a benefit from adjuvant 5-FU–based chemotherapy. However, this conclusion has been fraught with controversy, because the lack of benefit from 5-FU–based chemotherapy is not consistent across all studies evaluating MMR-D/MSI-H CRCs. 5-FU is a mainstay of chemotherapy for CRC in both the early stage and metastatic disease. In vitro studies have attempted to assess the effect of 5-FU on MSI-H CRC cell lines. Preclinical data using cell lines show that MMR-D cells seem to have a growth advantage and are more resistant to the cytotoxic effects of 5-FU compared with MMR-P cells.[37,38] Moreover, if MMR function was restored via chromosome 3 transfer, then, the growth advantage in the presence of 5-FU was no longer present.[37,38] Conflicting data showed that MMR-D cell lines, specifically, LOVO, showed similar sensitivity to 5-FU as MMR-D cell lines, SW480.[39] Subsequent evaluations of the MSI-H LOVO cell line showed increased thymidylate synthase activity and reduced sensitivity to 5-FU.[40] Data are also starting to emerge that the underlying cause of the MSI-H phenotype may be relevant in predicting response to 5-FU. For example, it has been suggested that MSI-H tumors with a CpG island methylator phenotype may show specific sensitivity to 5-FU.[41]

Initial clinical studies[42,43] evaluating response to 5-FU in MMR-D/MSI-H CRCs indicated a beneficial impact of 5-FU on stage III colon cancers with improved overall or recurrence-free survivals. However, the sample size was limited in both of these studies. A pivotal study published by Ribic and colleagues[34] analyzed patients with stage II and III colon cancer from pooled randomized clinical trials in which patients received either 5-FU chemotherapy or no treatment after surgical resection. Of 570 patients with tissue available, 95 had an MSI-H tumor, 53 of whom received 5-FU chemotherapy.[34] In the MSI-H patients who did not receive chemotherapy, an improved 5-year survival rate was reported; however, this survival advantage was not present in the MSI-H group who received 5-FU chemotherapy. Moreover, the study seemed to suggest that MSI-H patients with colon cancer who received 5-FU had a reduced survival compared with those who did not receive treatment. In an effort to provide validation of these findings, an international collaboration was formed to pool data from patients with stage II/III colon cancer receiving adjuvant 5-FU versus surgery alone as part of 5 different adjuvant colon cancer clinical trials.[44] Of the 457 patients, 70 (15%) had MMR-D/MSI-H colon cancer.[44] Although adjuvant 5-FU significantly improved disease-free survival (DFS) in the MSS/MMR-P tumors, in the MMR-D/MSI-H tumors receiving 5-FU, no improvement in DFS was seen.[44] When this data set (n = 457) and the Ribic data set (n = 570) were pooled, in the 515 untreated patients with stage II and III CRC, those with MMR-D/MSI-H had a clear improved

5-year DFS over MSS tumors. On the other hand, in the 512 treated patients with CRC, the improvement in DFS within the MMR-D/MSI-H subgroup was no longer apparent, suggesting that 5-FU may have abrogated the benefit associated with the MMR-D/MSI-H phenotype. Moreover, in patients with stage II colon cancer with MMR-D/MSI-H tumors, a reduced overall survival was seen (HR, 2.95; 95% CI, 1.02–8.54; P = .04).[44] The findings of a potential detrimental effect of 5-FU in MMR-D/MSI-H cases were specific to patients with stage II disease only, and applicability to other stages may not be appropriate.

Despite the data from these trials, there have been additional studies, including an analysis of patients treated in adjuvant colon cancer trials conducted by the National Surgery Adjuvant Breast and Bowel Project (NSABP), which reported no interaction between MMR status and 5-FU response.[35] Although an advantage of this trial was that MSI analysis was performed in a uniform way with the NCI-based reference of 5 markers, only 20% of all patients enrolled in the NSABP C-01 to C-04 studies had paraffin blocks that were suitable for MSI analysis.[35] In a more recent analysis including more then 600 patients with stage II/III colon cancer treated with 5-FU in the control arm of the Pan European Trial Adjuvant Colon Cancer (PETACC-3) study, a significant improvement in 5-year DFS was seen with MMR-D/MSI-H compared with MSS tumors, indicating that perhaps the improved prognosis is maintained even under 5-FU treatment.[45,46] Further analysis of this data set suggested that the prognostic impact of MSI-H phenotype is substantially stronger in stage II as opposed to stage III patients.[47] This finding may suggest stage-specific biological effects of the MMR-D/MSI-H phenotype. In contrast to the previous reports, in this study, the prognostic effect of MMR-D/MSI-H remained significant, despite treatment with 5-FU even in the stage II setting.

Adding to the evidence is a recent study by Sinicrope and colleagues,[48] who assessed stage II/III colon cancers and MMR status using samples from patients enrolled in adjuvant therapy clinical trials evaluating 5-FU with levamisole or leucovorin versus surgery alone. MMR-D/MSI-H was associated with reduced recurrence rates, delayed time to recurrence, and fewer distant recurrences. Distant recurrences were reduced with 5-FU–based adjuvant treatment in stage III but not in stage II MMR-D/MSI-H patients. Again, this finding seems to suggest that stage III colon cancers with MMR-D/MSI-H seem to benefit from 5-FU–based adjuvant treatment and should be treated with adjuvant chemotherapy per the current standard of care. In a subgroup analysis,[48] this study also suggested that any treatment benefit was restricted to patients with suspected germline as opposed to sporadic MMR-D/MSI-H. Studies assessing the response of MMR-D/MSI-H tumors to FOLFOX (5-FU, leucovorin, oxaliplatin) are awaited and may provide further insight into the outcome and the optimal treatment of MMR-D/MSI-H tumors.

Evidence overwhelmingly suggests that MMR-D/MSI-H CRC carries a better prognosis, yet, the efficacy of 5-FU chemotherapy in this subtype of CRC has been called into question. Bearing in mind the conflicting data, our general approach to the treatment of MMR-D/MSI-H CRC in the adjuvant setting has been that of avoiding the administration of 5-FU alone. Specifically, given the improved prognosis, as well as the lack of clear benefit (and suggestion of a potential detrimental effect), in stage II MMR-D/MSI-H CRCs, adjuvant treatment can generally be spared. In stage III MMR-D/MSI-H CRCs, there is no evidence to suggest that standard oxaliplatin-based treatment is ineffective, although the prognostic impact of MMR-D may be more modest in stage III as opposed to stage II CRCs. Our approach within the stage III setting has been to administer standard adjuvant treatment with an oxaliplatin-containing regimen. Studies assessing the response of MMR-D/MSI-H tumors to FOLFOX

(5-FU, leucovorin, oxaliplatin) are awaited and may provide further insight into the outcome and the optimal treatment of MMR-D/MSI-H tumors.

Irinotecan

Preclinical data also suggest that MMR-D/MSI-H CRC cell lines may be more sensitive to irinotecan, a topoisomerase I inhibitor, with known clinical efficacy in advanced CRC. Irinotecan introduces double-strand DNA breaks usually repaired by either homologous recombination or nonhomologous end joining. In tumors with MMR-D, mutations arising in microsatellite repeats in more than 30 genes have been described. Colorectal tumors and cell lines with MMR-D frequently accumulate mutations within microsatellite repeats of genes implicated in the double-strand DNA break repair pathway, including the MRE11A and hRAD50 genes. A mutation in either one of these genes results in significantly decreased expression of the Mre11/Nbs1/Rad50 (or MRN) protein complex. Mutations in MRE11 lead to a weak interaction with RAD50 and low affinity to Nbs1, compared with wild-type MRE11.[49,50] It has been postulated that decreased expression of the MRN protein complex leading to impaired double-stranded DNA break repair pathway in MMR-D tumors/cell lines may make these cells especially sensitive to agents that lead to disruption of DNA repair, such as irinotecan and potentially poly(ADP-ribose) polymerase inhibitors. MMR-D colon cancer cell lines that show an intronic frameshift mutation of MRE11 show the greatest sensitivity to irinotecan.[50,51]

In the clinical setting, the evidence for the impact of MMR-D/MSI-H on irinotecan sensitivity remains limited. In a retrospective analysis of 73 patients with metastatic CRC receiving second-line irinotecan-based therapy, a higher response rate was observed in MSI-H than in MSI-low or MSS tumors.[52] DFS according to MSI status was assessed through a retrospective evaluation of the Cancer and Leukemia Group B (CALGB) 89803 adjuvant trial,[53] which assigned patients with resected stage III colon cancer to 5-FU/leucovorin with or without irinotecan. Although in the overall group, no advantage for the addition of irinotecan to 5-FU/leucovorin was shown, in patients with MMR-D tumors, irinotecan resulted in a modest improvement in DFS.[53] The third study, presented at ASCO 2009, reported conflicting results.[45] In a retrospective analysis of the PETACC-3 trial, randomizing patients with stage II and III colon cancer to folinic acid, 5-FU, and irinotecan versus biweekly infusional 5-FU and folinic acid, of the 188 MSI-H cases, those treated with irinotecan did not have an improved survival. In a retrospective analysis of the Capecitabine, Irinotecan, and Oxaliplatin in advanced colorectal cancer (CAIRO) trial,[54] which included sequential irinotecan-containing treatments for metastatic CRC, the MSI-H cases were limited to only 14 and because both treatment arms received irinotecan at some point, interpretation of the MSI-H data was not possible. More studies to clarify the role of irinotecan in MSI-H cancers are clearly necessary. At this point, the use of irinotecan should be limited to advanced/metastatic CRC, irrespective of MMR status, because there is insufficient evidence for its use in the adjuvant setting, even in MMR-D/MSI-H tumors.

SUMMARY

The identification of the MMR-D/MSI-H subtype of CRC has important clinical implications for the prognosis of CRC, prediction of response to chemotherapeutic agents, specifically efficacy of 5-FU, and for the need for genetic assessment for Lynch syndrome. Recent expert consensus recommendations[20–22] suggest that either all patients with CRC or those with CRC at younger than 70 years, should undergo testing by either IHC or MSI, thereby leading to more patients with CRC being recognized as having this subtype of tumor. There is a pressing need for unambiguous answers with respect to the prognostic and predictive impact of MMR-D/MSI-H. Provocative, but preliminary, data suggesting a stage-specific impact and possible inherent biological differences between sporadic versus germline MMR-D/MSI-H tumors remain important questions awaiting validation.[47,48] With advances in gene expression profiling, next-generation sequencing technologies, and microRNA assessments, further biologically relevant classifications of CRC are anticipated, with MMR-D/MSI-H being just one of many relevant subgroups. Drug development and clinical trial design centered on specific molecular subtypes of tumors is a rapidly emerging approach to novel oncological treatments, and the MMR-D/MSI-H subtype may prove to be a useful marker for such targeted approaches.

REFERENCES

1. Ionov Y, Peinado MA, Malkhosyan S, et al. Ubiquitous somatic mutations in simple repeated sequences reveal a new mechanism for colonic carcinogenesis. Nature 1993;363:558–61.
2. Peltomaki P. Role of DNA mismatch repair defects in the pathogenesis of human cancer. J Clin Oncol 2003;21:1174–9.
3. Thibodeau SN, Bren G, Schaid D. Microsatellite instability in cancer of the proximal colon. Science 1993;260:816–9.
4. Hampel H, Frankel WL, Martin E, et al. Feasibility of screening for Lynch syndrome among patients with colorectal cancer. J Clin Oncol 2008;26:5783–8.
5. Hampel H, Frankel W, Panescu J, et al. Screening for Lynch syndrome (hereditary nonpolyposis colorectal cancer) among endometrial cancer patients. Cancer Res 2006;66:7810–7.
6. Fearon ER, Vogelstein B. A genetic model for colorectal tumorigenesis. Cell 1990;61:759–67.
7. Lengauer C, Kinzler KW, Vogelstein B. Genetic instabilities in human cancers. Nature 1998;396:643–9.
8. Lengauer C, Kinzler KW, Vogelstein B. Genetic instability in colorectal cancers. Nature 1997;386:623–7.
9. Eshleman JR, Casey JR, Kochera G, et al. Chromosome number and structure both are markedly stable in RER colorectal cancers and are not destabilized by mutation of p53. Oncogene 1998;17:719–25.
10. Herman JG, Umar A, Polyak K, et al. Incidence and functional consequences of hMLH1 promoter hypermethylation in colorectal carcinoma. Proc Natl Acad Sci U S A 1998;95:6870–5.
11. Kane MF, Loda M, Gaida GM, et al. Methylation of the hMLH1 promoter correlates with lack of expression of hMLH1 in sporadic colon tumors and mismatch repair-defective human tumor cell lines. Cancer Res 1997;57:808–11.
12. Jarvinen HJ, Aarnio M, Mustonen H, et al. Controlled 15-year trial on screening for colorectal cancer in families with hereditary nonpolyposis colorectal cancer. Gastroenterology 2000;118:829–34.
13. Vasen HF, Watson P, Mecklin JP, et al. New clinical criteria for hereditary nonpolyposis colorectal cancer (HNPCC, Lynch syndrome) proposed by the International Collaborative group on HNPCC. Gastroenterology 1999;116:1453–6.
14. Umar A, Boland CR, Terdiman JP, et al. Revised Bethesda Guidelines for hereditary nonpolyposis colorectal cancer (Lynch syndrome) and microsatellite instability. J Natl Cancer Inst 2004;96:261–8.
15. Julie C, Tresallet C, Brouquet A, et al. Identification in daily practice of patients with Lynch syndrome (hereditary nonpolyposis colorectal cancer): revised

Bethesda guidelines-based approach versus molecular screening. Am J Gastro-enterol 2008;103:2825–35 [quiz: 2836].

16. Canard G, Lefevre JH, Colas C, et al. Screening for Lynch syndrome in colorectal cancer: are we doing enough? Ann Surg Oncol 2012;19:809–16.

17. Leenen CH, van Lier MG, van Doorn HC, et al. Prospective evaluation of molecular screening for Lynch syndrome in patients with endometrial cancer </= 70 years. Gynecol Oncol 2012;125:414–20.

18. Mvundura M, Grosse SD, Hampel H, et al. The cost-effectiveness of genetic testing strategies for Lynch syndrome among newly diagnosed patients with colorectal cancer. Genet Med 2010;12:93–104.

19. Ladabaum U, Wang G, Terdiman J, et al. Strategies to identify the Lynch syndrome among patients with colorectal cancer: a cost-effectiveness analysis. Ann Intern Med 2011;155:69–79.

20. Vasen HF, Mecklin JP, Khan PM, et al. Revised guidelines for the clinical management of Lynch syndrome (HNPCC): recommendations by a group of European experts. Gut 2013;62:812–23.

21. Evaluation of Genomic Applications in Practice and Prevention (EGAPP) Working Group. Recommendations from the EGAPP Working Group: genetic testing strategies in newly diagnosed individuals with colorectal cancer aimed at reducing morbidity and mortality from Lynch syndrome in relatives. Genet Med 2009;11:35–41.

22. NCCN Genetic/Familial High-Risk Assessment: Colorectal (Version 2.2014). 2014. Available at: http://www.nccn.org/professionals/physician_gls/pdf/genetics_colon.pdf. Accessed November 3, 2014.

23. Cragun D, DeBate RD, Hampel H, et al. Comparing universal Lynch syndrome tumor-screening programs to evaluate associations between implementation strategies and patient follow-through. Genet Med 2014;16(10):773–82.

24. Boland CR, Thibodeau SN, Hamilton SR, et al. A National Cancer Institute Workshop on microsatellite instability for cancer detection and familial predisposition: development of international criteria for the determination of microsatellite instability in colorectal cancer. Cancer Res 1998;58:5248–57.

25. Rodriguez-Bigas MA, Boland CR, Hamilton SR, et al. A National Cancer Institute Workshop on hereditary nonpolyposis colorectal cancer syndrome: meeting highlights and Bethesda guidelines. J Natl Cancer Inst 1997;89:1758–62.

26. Zhang L. Immunohistochemistry versus microsatellite instability testing for screening colorectal cancer patients at risk for hereditary nonpolyposis colorectal cancer syndrome. Part II. The utility of microsatellite instability testing. J Mol Diagn 2008;10:301–7.

27. Shia J. Immunohistochemistry versus microsatellite instability testing for screening colorectal cancer patients at risk for hereditary nonpolyposis colorectal cancer syndrome. Part I. The utility of immunohistochemistry. J Mol Diagn 2008;10:293–300.

28. Oliveira C, Seruca R, Seixas M, et al. BRAF mutations characterize colon but not gastric cancer with mismatch repair deficiency. Oncogene 2003;22:9192–6.

29. Domingo E, Laiho P, Ollikainen M, et al. BRAF screening as a low-cost effective strategy for simplifying HNPCC genetic testing. J Med Genet 2004;41:664–8.

30. Deng G, Bell I, Crawley S, et al. BRAF mutation is frequently present in sporadic colorectal cancer with methylated hMLH1, but not in hereditary nonpolyposis colorectal cancer. Clin Cancer Res 2004;10:191–5.

31. Bapat B, Lindor NM, Baron J, et al. The association of tumor microsatellite instability phenotype with family history of colorectal cancer. Cancer Epidemiol Biomarkers Prev 2009;18:967–75.

32. Popat S, Hubner R, Houlston RS. Systematic review of microsatellite instability and colorectal cancer prognosis. J Clin Oncol 2005;23:609–18.
33. Gryfe R, Kim H, Hsieh ET, et al. Tumor microsatellite instability and clinical outcome in young patients with colorectal cancer. N Engl J Med 2000;342:69–77.
34. Ribic CM, Sargent DJ, Moore MJ, et al. Tumor microsatellite-instability status as a predictor of benefit from fluorouracil-based adjuvant chemotherapy for colon cancer. N Engl J Med 2003;349:247–57.
35. Kim GP, Colangelo LH, Wieand HS, et al. Prognostic and predictive roles of high-degree microsatellite instability in colon cancer: a National Cancer Institute-National Surgical Adjuvant Breast and Bowel Project Collaborative Study. J Clin Oncol 2007;25:767–72.
36. Lamberti C, Lundin S, Bogdanow M, et al. Microsatellite instability did not predict individual survival of unselected patients with colorectal cancer. Int J Colorectal Dis 2007;22:145–52.
37. Carethers JM, Chauhan DP, Fink D, et al. Mismatch repair proficiency and in vitro response to 5-fluorouracil. Gastroenterology 1999;117:123–31.
38. Meyers M, Wagner MW, Hwang HS, et al. Role of the hMLH1 DNA mismatch repair protein in fluoropyrimidine-mediated cell death and cell cycle responses. Cancer Res 2001;61:5193–201.
39. Chen XX, Lai MD, Zhang YL, et al. Less cytotoxicity to combination therapy of 5-fluorouracil and cisplatin than 5-fluorouracil alone in human colon cancer cell lines. World J Gastroenterol 2002;8:841–6.
40. van Triest B, Pinedo HM, Blaauwgeers JL, et al. Prognostic role of thymidylate synthase, thymidine phosphorylase/platelet-derived endothelial cell growth factor, and proliferation markers in colorectal cancer. Clin Cancer Res 2000;6:1063–72.
41. Iacopetta B, Kawakami K, Watanabe T. Predicting clinical outcome of 5-fluorouracil-based chemotherapy for colon cancer patients: is the CpG island methylator phenotype the 5-fluorouracil-responsive subgroup? Int J Clin Oncol 2008;13: 498–503.
42. Elsaleh H, Joseph D, Grieu F, et al. Association of tumour site and sex with survival benefit from adjuvant chemotherapy in colorectal cancer. Lancet 2000; 355:1745–50.
43. Hemminki A, Mecklin JP, Jarvinen H, et al. Microsatellite instability is a favorable prognostic indicator in patients with colorectal cancer receiving chemotherapy. Gastroenterology 2000;119:921–8.
44. Sargent DJ, Marsoni S, Monges G, et al. Defective mismatch repair as a predictive marker for lack of efficacy of fluorouracil-based adjuvant therapy in colon cancer. J Clin Oncol 2010;28:3219–26.
45. Tejpar S, Bosman F, Delorenzi M, et al. Microsatellite instability (MSI) in stage II and III colon cancer treated with 5FU-LV or 5FU-LV and irinotecan (PETACC-3-EORTC 40993-SAKK 60/00 trial) [abstract]. J Clin Oncol 2009;27:a4001.
46. Tejpar S, Saridaki Z, Delorenzi M, et al. Microsatellite instability, prognosis and drug sensitivity of stage II and III colorectal cancer: more complexity to the puzzle. J Natl Cancer Inst 2011;103:841–4.
47. Roth AD, Tejpar S, Yan P, et al. Correlation of molecular markers in colon cancer with stage-specific prognosis: results of the translational study on the PETACC3-EORTC 40993-SAKK 60–00 trial. 2009 ASCO GI Cancer Symposium. San Francisco, CA, January 15–17, 2009. [abstract 288].
48. Sinicrope FA, Foster NR, Thibodeau SN, et al. DNA mismatch repair status and colon cancer recurrence and survival in clinical trials of 5-fluorouracil-based adjuvant therapy. J Natl Cancer Inst 2011;103:863–75.

49. Alemayehu A, Fridrichova I. The MRE11/RAD50/NBS1 complex destabilization in Lynch-syndrome patients. Eur J Hum Genet 2007;15:922–9.

50. Wen Q, Scorah J, Phear G, et al. A mutant allele of MRE11 found in mismatch repair-deficient tumor cells suppresses the cellular response to DNA replication fork stress in a dominant negative manner. Mol Biol Cell 2008;19:1693–705.

51. Rodriguez R, Hansen LT, Phear G, et al. Thymidine selectively enhances growth suppressive effects of camptothecin/irinotecan in MSI+ cells and tumors containing a mutation of MRE11. Clin Cancer Res 2008;14:5476–83.

52. Fallik D, Borrini F, Boige V, et al. Microsatellite instability is a predictive factor of the tumor response to irinotecan in patients with advanced colorectal cancer. Cancer Res 2003;63:5738–44.

53. Bertagnolli MM, Niedzwiecki D, Compton CC, et al. Microsatellite instability predicts improved response to adjuvant therapy with irinotecan, fluorouracil, and leucovorin in stage III colon cancer: Cancer and Leukemia Group B Protocol 89803. J Clin Oncol 2009;27:1814–21.

54. Koopman M, Kortman GA, Mekenkamp L, et al. Deficient mismatch repair system in patients with sporadic advanced colorectal cancer. Br J Cancer 2009;100: 266–73.

Predictive and Prognostic Markers in the Treatment of Metastatic Colorectal Cancer (mCRC): Personalized Medicine at Work

Sebastian Stintzing, MD, Stefan Stremitzer, MD, Ana Sebio, MD, Heinz-Josef Lenz, MD*

KEYWORDS

- Colorectal cancer • BRAF • KRAS • NRAS • Biomarker

KEY POINTS

- Extended RAS analysis, including mutations in KRAS exons 2, 3, and 4 and NRAS exons 2, 3, and 4, defines the subpopulation of patients that most likely benefit from anti–epidermal growth factor receptor treatment.
- RAS currently remains the only established predictive biomarker in the treatment of metastatic colorectal cancer (mCRC).
- BRAF mutations are the second biomarker that may be tested for.
- Patients with an excellent performance status and a BRAF mutant tumor can be considered for FOLFOXIRI (leucovorin, 5-fluorouracil, oxaliplatin, irinotecan) therapy, as this has shown remarkable outcomes in a small phase II trial in patients bearing a BRAF mutant tumor.
- The mechanisms of action of anti–vascular endothelial growth factor are too diversified, and no predictive factor has yet been identified or validated.

INTRODUCTION

Colorectal cancer (CRC) is one of the most frequent and deadliest cancers worldwide, with an estimated 136,830 new cases and an estimated 50,310 deaths in 2014 in the United States.[1] Survival times in metastatic disease have significantly improved over

The authors declare no conflict of interest.
Funding: Supported by the 5P30CA014089-27S1 grant, and the Daniel Butler Research Fund. S. Stintzing is supported by a postdoctoral fellowship from the German Cancer Aid (Mildred-Scheel Foundation, grant number 110422). S. Stremitzer is a recipient of an Erwin Schrödinger fellowship. A. Sebio is a recipient of a Rio Hortega Research Grant from the Insituto de Salud Carlos III (CM11/00102).
Sharon Carpenter Laboratory, University of Southern California/Norris Comprehensive Cancer Center, Keck School of Medicine, 1441 Eastlake Avenue, Room 3456, Los Angeles, CA 90033, USA
* Corresponding author.
E-mail address: lenz@usc.edu

Hematol Oncol Clin N Am 29 (2015) 43–60
http://dx.doi.org/10.1016/j.hoc.2014.09.009
0889-8588/15/$ – see front matter © 2015 Elsevier Inc. All rights reserved.

the past several decades, lately reaching 24 to 30 months in clinical trials.[2,3] However, 5-year survival rates remain at a low of about 8%.[4] The therapeutic regimen evolved from single-agent 5-fluorouracil (5-FU), with response rates of about 20% to 25%, to chemotherapeutic combination of leucovorin and 5-FU with oxaliplatin (FOLFOX) or irinotecan (FOLFIRI), with response rates of around 40% to 55%.[5,6] Infusional 5-FU can be substituted by the rational designed drug capecitabine, which is a prodrug to 5-FU.[7] In metastatic CRC (mCRC), most therapeutic regimens are based on 5-FU. Combination regimens such as FOLFIRI and FOLFOX reach median overall survival (OS) times of about 20 months.[5] During the 2000s, the introduction of antibody treatment against the vascular endothelial growth factor (VEGF) using bevacizumab and the epidermal growth factor receptor (EGFR) using cetuximab or panitumumab has further increased response rates and survival times.[2,8–10] The antiangiogenic treatment principle has, in addition to the VEGF-A antibody bevacizumab, guided the development of aflibercept, a recombinant fusion protein to target VEGF-A, VEGF-B, and placental growth factor (PIGF). The multikinase inhibitor regorafenib is also targeting angiogenesis and has a relative specificity to VEGF receptors 1 to 3, platelet-derived growth factor receptor (PDGFR), and other protein kinases.[11] Regorafenib statistically significantly prolonged survival by 1.4 months in a phase III placebo-controlled trial, and is approved for further-line treatment of mCRC.[12] The VELOUR study demonstrated efficacy for aflibercept in combination with FOLFIRI in second-line treatment of mCRC after FOLFOX failure by statistically significantly prolonging survival by 1.4 months.[13] For a selected patient population with younger age and good performance status, trials suggest that a combination of leucovorin, 5-FU, irinotecan, and oxaliplatin (FOLFOXIRI) may further extend the survival benefit reached by cytotoxic agents in mCRC.[14]

The development of new drugs and the introduction of combination regimens have prolonged survival from 6 months to 24 to 30 months. The decision made in selection of first-line treatment is important for OS, but current guidelines are rather nonspecific and offer a panoply of possibilities.[15] In recent years it has become increasingly clear that certain subpopulations of mCRC may derive significant advantage from targeted treatments, whereas other patients do not benefit or might even be harmed by certain combinations. As technologies such as next-generation sequencing (NGS)-based screening for mutations and polymorphism and gene-expression arrays become more accessible, new prognostic and predictive subpopulations of mCRC will be defined. This advance will open up new opportunities to predict treatment response, resistance, and toxicity, and will stimulate drug development by defining novel druggable targets. Approaches such as liquid biopsies will further help to achieve a better understanding of the development of treatment resistance and the best treatment sequence for the individual patient.

PREDICTIVE BIOMARKERS FOR ANTI–EPIDERMAL GROWTH FACTOR RECEPTOR
The Rat Sarcoma Story

As of now, the only established and widely accepted predictive biomarker in the treatment of mCRC is mutation of the RAS proto-oncogene.[16] The anti-EGFR antibodies cetuximab and panitumumab have been shown to prolong survival in further-line treatment when applied as monotherapy[17,18] or in combination with irinotecan.[19] The predictive value of KRAS exon 2 (codons 12 and 13) mutations for cetuximab was first described in a small retrospective analysis of 30 treated patients.[20] The first-line phase III trial testing FOLFIRI plus cetuximab against FOLFIRI alone (CRYSTAL study) confirmed the negative predictive value of KRAS exon 2 mutations for cetuximab treatment.[17] The phase II OPUS study testing FOLFOX against FOLFOX plus cetuximab was the first to reveal a potential harm regarding progression-free survival (PFS) and OS in patients with KRAS exon 2 mutant tumors[9] treated with cetuximab. Accordingly the approval for cetuximab was subsequently restricted to KRAS exon 2 wild-type patients. The PRIME study, a first-line phase III study testing FOLFOX plus panitumumab versus FOLFOX, confirmed the negative predictive value of KRAS exon 2 mutations[10] for the use of panitumumab. All 3 studies showed improved efficacy for anti-EGFR plus chemotherapeutic treatment when compared with chemotherapy alone only in the KRAS exon 2 wild-type population.[9,10,17] Further analysis suggested that different mutations might have different predictive value and that exon 2 codon 13 (p.G13D) mutations might have a less detrimental effect on cetuximab treatment,[21,22] although numbers were too small to establish a clear conclusion.

With further analyses of the PRIME study it has become clear that all RAS mutations, including not only all KRAS exon 2 but also KRAS mutations within exon 3 (codons 59 and 61) and exon 4 (codons 117 and 146), in addition to mutations within the NRAS (neuroblastoma RAS) exon 2 (codons 12 and 13), exon 3 (exons 59 and 61), and exon 4 (codons 117 and 146), were more frequent in mCRC than previously described[23] and, when combined, have a negative predictive value comparable with what has been seen in KRAS exon 2 mutant tumors.[24] NRAS shares more than 90% of the KRAS protein and has similar functions.[25] The extended RAS analysis revealed another 8% to 35% of RAS (KRAS and NRAS) mutations within the KRAS exon 2 wild-type population (**Fig. 1**).[24,26–28] The population defined by the extended RAS analysis as "RAS wild-type" had a statistically significant OS benefit when treated with panitumumab and FOLFOX in comparison with FOLFOX alone, and the hazard ratio in favor for the panitumumab arm improved from 0.83 to 0.78.[24,29] The influence of the extended RAS analyses on study end points of the OPUS, PEAK, FIRE-3, PICCOLO, and CORE-2 studies are summarized in **Table 1**. As a consequence of these data, the use of anti-EGFR antibodies in mCRC is now restricted to RAS wild-type patients.

It is important to mention that different detection methods have different sensitivities, leading to different frequencies of RAS mutations. The methods used are Sanger-Sequencing, with a sensitivity of 10% to 20%,[30] Pyrosequencing, with a sensitivity of less than 5%,[31] WAVE based SURVEYOR Scan Kits (Transgenomic, Omaha,

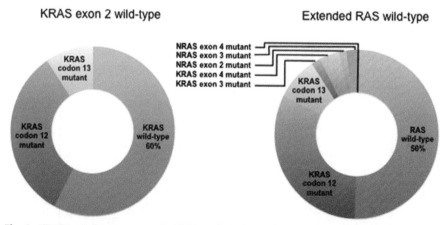

Fig. 1. KRAS exon 2 versus extended RAS analysis. (*Data from* Douillard JY, Oliner KS, Siena S, et al. Panitumumab-FOLFOX4 treatment and RAS mutations in colorectal cancer. N Engl J Med 2013;369(11):1023–34.)

Table 1
Studies published with extended RAS analyses using cetuximab/panitumumab in the treatment of metastatic colorectal cancer

Trial (KRASwt)(RASwt)	Treatment Arms	ORR (%)	P* OR	ORR (%) Extended RAS	P* OR	PFS (mo)	P** HR	PFS (mo) Extended RAS	P** HR	OS (mo)	P** HR	OS (mo) Extended RAS	P** HR
First-Line Treatment													
PRIME													
n = 656	FOLFOX	48	.068	NA	NA	8.0	.02	7.9	.004	19.4	.03	20.2	.009
n = 512	FOLFOX + Pan	55	1.35			9.6	0.80	10.1	0.72	23.8	0.82	25.8	0.78
OPUS													
n = 179	FOLFOX	34.0	.002	30.4	.008	7.2	.006	5.8	.018	18.5	.39	17.8	.50
n = 82	FOLFOX + Cet	57.3	2.55	61.1	3.46	8.3	0.57	12.0	0.43	22.8	0.86	20.7	0.83
FIRE-3													
n = 592	FOLFIRI + Cet	62.0	.18	65.5	.32	10.0	.547	10.4	.54	28.7	.017	33.1	.011
n = 342	FOLFIRI + Bev	58.0	1.18	59.6	1.28	10.3	1.06	10.2	0.93	25.0	0.77	25.6	0.70
PEAK													
n = 285	FOLFOX + Pan	58	NA	64	NA	10.9	.22	13.0	.03	34.2	.009	41.3	.06
n = 170	FOLFOX + Bev	54		60		10.1	0.84	10.1	0.66	24.3	0.62	28.9	0.63
CORE-2													
n = 152 / n = 124[a]	FOLFOX + Cet	57.9	NA	61.3[a]	NA	9.3	NA	9.7[a]	NA	25.2	NA	28.5[a]	NA
Second-Line Treatment													
PICCOLO													
n = 597	FOLFIRI	10	.001	12	NA	3.9	.004	NA	.015	12.5	.12	NA	.91
n = 323	FOLFIRI + Pan	35	NA	34	NA	5.9	0.73	NA	0.78	14.5	0.85	NA	1.01

Abbreviations: Bev, bevacizumab; Cet, cetuximab; HR, hazard ratio; KRASwt, number of patients with KRAs exon 2 wild-type tumors; NA, not available; OR, odds ratio; ORR, overall response rate; OS, overall survival; P*, Fisher's exact test P; P**, log-rank test P; Pan, panitumumab; PFS, progression-free survival; RASwt, number of patients with extended RAS analyses wild-type tumors.

[a] In CORE-2 study, data for RAS and BRAF wild-type are given.

NE, USA), with a sensitivity of approximately 1%,[32] and BEAMing technology (Sysmex Inostics, Inc, Baltimore, MD, USA), with a sensitivity of 0.01%.[33] To date no cutoff analysis has been presented, and the question remains as to at what level of detection sensitivity patients will still benefit from anti-EGFR treatment. The detection of 0.1% or 0.01% RAS mutations may be critical to identify subclones that will outgrow anti-EGFR therapy but may be not sufficient to withhold therapy.[34] For the analyses of KRAS exon 2 (codons 12 and13) a sensitivity between 1% and 5% has been regarded as sufficient. The widely used cobas KRAS mutation test (Roche Molecular Diagnostics, Pleasanton, CA, USA) has a sensitivity of less than 5%.[35] The only test for KRAS exon 2 (codon 12 and 13) approved by the Food and Drug Administration has a sensitivity of 1% (TheraScreen KRAS test; Qiagen, Valencia, CA, USA).[36]

Recently it has been suggested that RAS mutations may have a predictive value for the use of oxaliplatin in first-line treatment of mCRC, as RAS mutant patients in one report had a longer PFS and OS when compared with RAS wild-type patients.[37] Cell culture experiments revealed a higher efficacy for oxaliplatin in KRAS mutation transfected colorectal cancer cell lines by downregulating ERCC1 levels.[38] In a German AIO study comparing CAPIRI (capecitabine plus irinotecan) against CAPOX (capecitabine plus oxaliplatin) both in combination with bevacizumab in first-line treatment of mCRC, a statistically significantly longer OS of the irinotecan arm in KRAS exon 2 mutant patients was demonstrated.[39] More data are needed to better understand the role of RAS mutations and their chemosensitivity to oxaliplatin.

Other Mutations in the Epidermal Growth Factor Receptor Signaling Pathway

The relations and positions of the different predictive and prognostic markers in the EGFR-dependent signaling cascade are illustrated in **Fig. 2**.

BRAF

BRAF is a member of the RAF (RAS-associated factor) gene family, which is downstream of RAS. Activating BRAF mutations (exon 15, V600E) are detected in about 10% to 15% of all mCRC cases.[40] mCRC cases with both RAS and BRAF mutations are extremely rare, with an estimated frequency of 0.001%.[27,41] Patients with BRAF mutant tumors have a poor prognosis, with short median OS times ranging from 9 to 14 months.[2,42–44] Because of the small numbers of patients in individual trials, pooled analyses using data from several randomized trials were performed to determine the prognostic and/or predictive value of BRAF mutant tumors in patients with mCRC.[2] Even then, no statistically significant statement could be made. However, there is a consensus that BRAF mutations are prognostic markers. There are data suggesting that patients with BRAF mutant mCRC may still benefit from first-line anti-EGFR therapy; however, some of the best clinical outcome data in these patients was shown using FOLFOXIRI plus bevacizumab in first-line treatment, reaching 11.8 months of PFS and 24.1 months of OS.[45] Single-agent BRAF inhibitors have shown clinical efficacy in other tumor entities, but in mCRC single-agent activity was low. However, the combination of BRAF inhibitors and anti-EGFR antibodies is looking promising because of upregulated EGFR expression.

PIK3CA mutations

Phosphatidylinositol-4,5-bisphosphate 3-kinase catalytic subunit α (PIK3CA) is subordinate to RAS and BRAF, activated through EGFR signaling (see **Fig. 2**). PIK3CA mutations can be detected in about 10% to 30% of mCRC samples.[46] In almost 50% of cases, PIK3CA mutant tumors also harbor a concomitant BRAF mutation[47,48] and in about 40% another RAS mutation[41,49] (**Fig. 3**), which makes it difficult to assess the

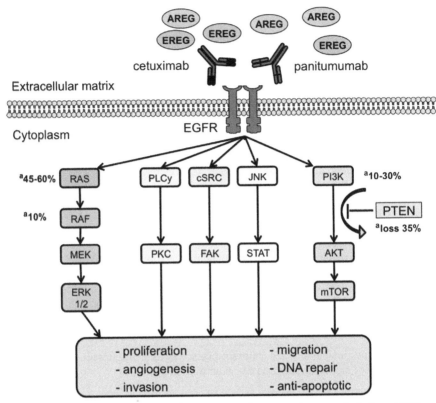

Fig. 2. Simplified EGFR signaling pathway. AKT, AKR mouse thymoma inducing; AREG, amphiregulin; cSRC, cellular sarcoma inducing; EGFR, epithelial growth factor receptor; EREG, epiregulin; ERK, extracellular signal–regulated kinases; FAK, focal adhesion kinase; JNK, janus kinase; MEK, mitogen-activated protein kinase; mTOR, mammalian target of rapamycin; PI3K, phosphatidylinositol-3-kinase; PKC, protein kinase C; PLCy, phospholipase C; PTEN, phosphatase and tensin homologue; RAF, RAS-associated factor; RAS, rat sarcoma; STAT, signal transducer and activator of transcription. [a] Frequency of mutations in mCRC.

predictive and prognostic value. PIK3CA mutations in CRC have gained more attention since a report claimed a higher survival rate in PIK3CA mutant adjuvant CRC patients taking aspirin,[50] although a recently presented study was not able to confirm this.[51]

After excluding all cases with concomitant RAS and BRAF mutations, PIK3CA mutations were shown to have an influence on survival times in 649 patients treated with cetuximab plus chemotherapy in a pooled analysis of chemotherapy-refractory patients.[52] As no cetuximab-free control arm was tested, it remains unclear whether the value is predictive or prognostic. As PIK3CA and mTOR inhibitors have been developed, it might be worthwhile to test the effect of these drugs in combination with an anti-EGFR strategy in patients bearing a PIK3CA mutation which are otherwise RAS and BRAF wild-type.[53]

In mCRC, codon 9 and codon 20 mutations in PIK3CA have been described, and the predictive value may be limited to codon 20 mutations only.[54] Furthermore, PI3KCA signaling is activated through the phosphorylated intracellular domain of receptor tyrosine kinases or by RAS oncogenes and even estrogen.[55] Embedded into such

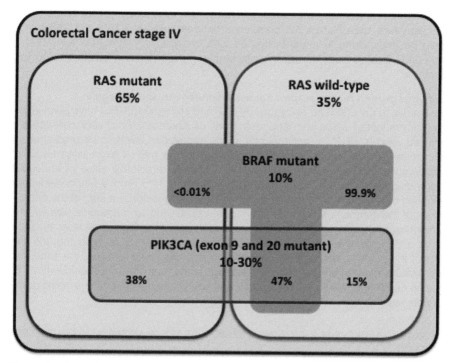

Fig. 3. Overlap of mutations in colorectal cancer. (*Data from* Refs.[41,49] and Stintzing S, Jung A, Rossius L, et al. Mutations within the EGFR signaling pathway: influence on efficacy in FIRE-3–A randomized phase III study of FOLFIRI plus cetuximab or bevacizumab as first-line treatment for wild-type (WT) KRAS (exon 2) metastatic colorectal cancer (mCRC) patients. J Clin Oncol 2014;32(Suppl 3) [abstract: 445].)

an interconnected and redundant network, the prognostic value of isolated PIK3CA mutations is difficult to assess, and as yet no clinical usefulness for testing for PIK3CA mutations in mCRC has been demonstrated.

Phosphatase and tensin homologue expression/mutations

Phosphatase and tensin homologue (PTEN) is an inhibitor of PIK3CA signaling. In CRC, PTEN is inactivated in 20% to 30% because of epigenetic/genetic mechanisms, such as hypermethylation and mutations or loss of heterozygosity.[56] Immunohisto-chemical staining reveals a loss of PTEN in up to 35% of CRC cases.[57] There is also a correlation between microsatellite instability (MSI) tumors and PTEN alterations because about 30% of MSI tumors, but only 9% of microsatellite-stable tumors, harbor PTEN mutations.[58] The prognostic value of PTEN loss and mutations remains unclear, as multiple studies have used different detection methods and different end points.

Multiple studies investigated the possible predictive value of PTEN loss in patients treated with the anti-EGFR antibodies cetuximab and panitumumab. Most of them used immunohistochemistry for detection. Some smaller studies were able to find a negative prognostic value for cetuximab and panitumumab.[59] Others were able to demonstrate different predictive values of PTEN expression in metastases when compared with primary tumor tissue.[60] The largest cohort of tumor tissue from a randomized trial derives from the CAIRO-2 study, in which 559 tumor samples were investigated. No correlation between loss of PTEN and PFS or OS could be established in patients treated with cetuximab.[61] The data for PTEN in anti-EGFR–treated patients are inconsistent, but thus far no predictive value can be stated.

Epidermal growth factor receptor ligands amphiregulin and epiregulin

The ligands to the EGFR amphiregulin (AREG) and epiregulin (EREG) have been intensively investigated since the landmark work of Khambata-Ford and colleagues[62] revealed, next to KRAS mutational status, the expression levels to be predictive for cetuximab efficacy. Multiple studies investigating the mRNA expression levels of amphiregulin and epiregulin were able to confirm the predictive value of epiregulin and/or epiregulin levels for cetuximab-treated patients.[63–65] From a functional standpoint this makes perfect sense, as a higher ligand expression is a sign of the dependence of the tumor cells on the EGFR pathway. Owing to methodical issues, the transformation into clinical practice has not been possible so far. Expression measurements depend on the accuracy of how the tumor cells have been collected, the efficacy of the primer pairs used for real-time polymerase chain reaction, the annealing temperature the choice of the housekeeping genes, and the cutoff calculation. To date no cutoff and measurement method has been established, and it remains questionable whether these challenges can be overcome.

PREDICTIVE MARKERS FOR ANTIANGIOGENIC THERAPY IN METASTATIC COLORECTAL CANCER

Antiangiogenic drugs are widely used, and target the VEGF signaling pathway. Bevacizumab, the first-in-class drug, targets VEGF-A and prevents VEGF from binding to its receptors. Aflibercept binds both VEGF isoforms (A and B) and PIGF, a ligand that has been postulated as a potential cause of bevacizumab resistance.[66] These drugs are not cytotoxic, but modulate the tumor environment and decrease tumor neoangiogenesis. As these agents do not target tumor cells, efforts aimed at finding predictive markers within tumor cells have failed thus far.[67] Pharmacogenetic approaches investigating genetic variations within VEGF-dependent pathways are more promising,[68] but as of now no predictive marker has been established. Circulating markers, such as the VEGF-independent proangiogenic factor interleukin-8[69] or plasma VEGF-A levels,[70] have shown promising predictive value in closely monitored preliminary studies. Because of difficulties in standardization of sample handling and challenging considerations regarding cutoffs of circulating markers, no predictive biomarker for antiangiogenic treatment has yet been established.

PREDICTIVE MARKERS FOR THE CHEMOTHERAPEUTIC BACKGROUND
5-Fluorouracil

5-FU remains the most used and most active drug in the treatment of mCRC. The antimetabolite 5-FU is a pyrimidine analogue that inhibits thymidylate synthase (TS) irreversibly. The successive lack of thymidine triphosphate inhibits DNA replication, resulting in cell death of rapid proliferative cells.[71] With the exception of the monotherapeutic use of regorafenib and anti-EGFR antibodies cetuximab or panitumumab in further-line treatment, all regimens contain 5-FU or one of the orally available 5-FU prodrugs capecitabine, UFT (tegafur/uracil), or S1 (tegafur/gimeracil/oteracil). 5-FU is metabolized more than 80% in the liver by dihydropyrimidine dehydrogenase

(DPD). TS and DPD have been extensively investigated in regard to their predictive value for 5-FU treatment.

A relative DPD deficiency with a higher possibility of grade 3/4 toxicity exists in 3% to 5% of patients, but a complete DPD deficiency causing serious adverse events is rare, with a frequency of 0.1%.[72] Single-nucleotide polymorphisms (SNPs) within the DPD are responsible for the variability of DPD activity and 5-FU toxicity.[73] Several studies demonstrated a correlation between DPD tumor expression and chemotherapeutic efficacy,[74,75] and recently it has been shown that SNPs within the DPD may also predict outcome.[76] However, as of now DPD is predictive for 5-FU toxicity rather than its efficacy.

TS is the primary target of 5-FU and has been extensively studied as a predictor for 5-FU efficacy. High intratumor TS expression was correlated with shorter OS in a large meta-analysis of 20 studies in both adjuvant and metastatic CRC.[77] Cutoff differences and unresolved challenges to implement sound cross-center stable measurements of intratumor RNA expression levels make a clinical implementation difficult. SNPs to the TS gene are another approach to investigate TS as a predictive marker. SNPs are easy, inexpensive, and quick to access. Several SNPs in the TS gene have been described to be of potentially predictive value,[78] but validation studies are lacking. To distinguish between the predictive and possible prognostic value of TS expression a control arm not containing 5-FU would be necessary, which is impossible to find in the treatment of mCRC.

No validated predictive marker for the use of 5-FU has been established as yet. DPD deficiency remains to be predictive for toxicity, although routine measurement of DPD is not current practice.

Oxaliplatin

Oxaliplatin forms inter-DNA and intra-DNA cross-links, which disrupt DNA replication and result in cell death.[79] Oxaliplatin has essentially no single-agent activity in mCRC but is used in a variety of combinations with 5-FU (FUFOX, FOLFOX)[80] or irinotecan (IrOx).[81] DNA cross-links can be removed by the base excision repair system. One of the key components representing the rate-limiting process of the excision repair system is the excision repair cross-complementing group 1 (ERCC1) enzyme. The data on ERCC1 intratumor expression and efficacy in oxaliplatin-based chemotherapy is contradictory. In one first-line study low ERCC1 expression was associated with longer survival[82]; however, the CAIRO study investigating 506 primary tumor samples in patients treated with oxaliplatin in second and third line after CAPIRI or capecitabine first-line therapy was unable to confirm this observation,[74] possibly because of changes in ERCC1 expression during first-line therapy. SNPs in ERCC1 have been tested for their predictive value but, again because of the lack of validation studies and controls, none has made it into clinical practice.[83] The importance of intratumor ERCC1 levels for oxaliplatin efficacy and resistance is underlined by data showing that ERCC1 and DPD is upregulated in CRC samples after oxaliplatin-based first-line therapy for mCRC.[84]

Recently the randomized phase II MAVERICC trial (NCT01374425), prospectively testing ERCC1 expression as a biomarker for FOLFIRI or FOLFOX first-line treatment of mCRC, has completed recruitment. With a planned recruitment of 360 patients, this will be the first study prospectively stratifying for a biomarker in the treatment of mCRC.

Detoxification of oxaliplatin depends on glutathione S-transferase family members. SNPs have been shown to be of predictive value for oxaliplatin-dependent

Table 2
Overview of important predictive and prognostic factors in the treatment of metastatic colorectal cancer (mCRC)

Pathway	Marker	Value	Clinical Conclusion
EGFR	RAS mutation in KRAS and NRAS Exon 2 (codons 12, 13) Exon 3 (codons 59, 61) Exon 4 (codons 117, 146)	Negative predictive for the use of cetuximab and panitumumab	Established biomarker in the treatment of mCRC
EGFR	BRAF mutation	Negative prognostic value Possible negative predictive value for cetuximab and panitumumab	FOLFOXIRI may be discussed in a certain subpopulation
EGFR	PIK3CA mutation	Negative predictive value for the use of cetuximab and panitumumab is discussed but not validated	Not a validated biomarker, no clinical conclusion
EGFR	PTEN loss PTEN mutations	Negative predictive value has been discussed for both mutations and loss of expression	Not a validated biomarker, no clinical conclusion
EGFR	AREG EREG	Higher expression levels are associated with increased response to anti-EGFR therapy with cetuximab	Methodological problems in measuring expression levels and cutoff calculations are ongoing. Not to be used in clinical practice
VEGF	VEGF-A plasma levels	Higher VEGF-A plasma levels predict increase in bevacizumab efficacy	Methodological problems. Not to be used in clinical practice
VEGF	IL-8	Bevacizumab predictor as a VEGF-A independent proangiogenic factor	Methodological problems. Not to be used in clinical practice
VEGF	SNP	Predictive VEGF SNPs and VEGFR SNPs for bevacizumab.	Easy to measure but not validated. Not to be used in clinical practice
TS	TS expression	Predictive for 5-FU. Higher TS expression correlated significant in adjuvant and mCRC with shorter OS	Methodological problems. Not to be used in clinical practice. A 5-FU–free control arm is difficult to create
DPD	DPD deficiency	Complete deficiency is rare (0.1%) but even relative deficiency due to polymorphisms (3%–5%) are predictive for 5-FU toxicity	Screening is not recommended

(continued on next page)

Table 2
(continued)

Pathway	Marker	Value	Clinical Conclusion
BER	ERCC1 expression level	ERCC1 expression levels are predictive for oxaliplatin response in first-line treatment. Data on second and third-line treatment was inconclusive.	Results from a prospective randomized phase II trial are awaited. Not to be used in clinical practice as yet
GSTP1	SNP	SNPs have been predictive for oxaliplatin induced neurotoxicity	Easy to measure but not validated. Not to be used in clinical practice
TOPO1	TOPO1 expression	Higher TOPO1 expression has been associated with longer OS in irinotecan and oxaliplatin-treated patients	Methodological problems. Not to be used in clinical practice
UGT1A1	UGT1A1 SNPs	Genetic variations of UGT1A1 are predictive for irinotecan toxicity	Test is recommended in the USA. Regimen with lower irinotecan dosing do not have UGT1A1-related toxicity problems
Ataxin	APTX expression	APTX is involved in repairing irinotecan-related DNA strand breaks	Not validated in a trial with a higher number of patients. Not to be used in clinical practice

Abbreviations: 5-FU, 5-fluorouracil; APTX, ataxin; AREG, amphiregulin; DPD, dihydropyrimidine dehydrogenase; EGFR, epidermal growth factor receptor; EREG, epiregulin; FOLFOXIRI, leucovorin, 5-FU, oxaliplatin, irinotecan; IL-8, interleukin-8; OS, overall survival; PTEN, phosphatase and tensin homologue; SNP, single-nucleotide polymorphism; TPO1, topoisomerase 1; TS, thymidylate synthase; UGT1A1, uridine diphosphate glucuronosyltransferase 1A1; VEGF, vascular endothelial growth factor; VEGFR, VEGF receptor.

neurotoxicity[83,85] and efficacy,[86,87] but again validation studies are lacking so the value for clinical decision making is unclear.

Irinotecan

Irinotecan is hydrolyzed to SN38, which is a topoisomerase 1 (TOPO1) inhibitor. Inhibition of TOPO1 leads to inhibition of DNA replication and transcription by inducing single- and double-strand breaks and DNA fragmentation. SN38 is detoxified by uridine diphosphate glucuronosyltransferase 1A1 (UGT1A1). Genetic variants of UGT1A1 are associated with enzyme activity and irinotecan toxicity in regimens using higher doses of irinotecan.[88] Irinotecan has shown single-agent activity after 5-FU failure,[89] but is usually administered in combination with anti-EGFR therapy[19] in further therapy lines or with 5-FU[5,90] in first-line and second-line regimens. Defined by the mechanism of action and detoxification, biomarker development has been focused on TOPO1 and UGT1A1.

In UGT1A1, owing to the known toxicity issues, research on the predictive value has focused on SNPs. However, published results have been controversial, and it is hypothesized that an SNP signature might be predictive for irinotecan use.[91,92]

The data on TOPO1 expression for prediction of irinotecan efficacy are controversial. The United Kingdom–based FOCUS trial tested 822 samples successfully for

TOPO1 expression by immunohistochemistry. A high TOPO1 expression was associated with a significantly longer survival in both irinotecan-treated and oxaliplatin-treated patients, with a higher predictive value for irinotecan-treated patients.[93] These data were confirmed in a smaller trial using fluorescence in situ hybridization,[94] but the association with oxaliplatin use is not understood and a prospective trial is needed.

Aprataxin (APTX) is a gene involved in the repair of DNA strand breaks[95] as caused by irinotecan. The immunohistochemical expression of APTX has suggested it to be of predictive value for irinotecan treatment in CRC,[96] but no confirmation study has been conducted thus far (**Table 2**).

SUMMARY

Extended RAS analysis, including mutations of KRAS exons 2, 3, and 4 and NRAS exons 2, 3, and 4, defines the subpopulation of patients that most likely benefit from anti-EGFR treatment. RAS currently remains the only established predictive biomarker in the treatment of mCRC. It only has negative predictive value, but should be assessed at first diagnosis of metastatic disease. BRAF mutations are the second biomarker that may be tested for. Patients with an excellent performance status and a BRAF mutant tumor can be considered for FOLFOXIRI therapy, as this has shown remarkable outcomes in a small phase II trial in patients bearing a BRAF mutant tumor. Several recent studies have suggested that gene-expression levels of EREG and AREG may be predictive biomarkers for EGFR inhibitors, although the validation and standardization of the technologies have limited the implementation of these biomarkers in the clinic. The mechanisms of action of anti-VEGF are too diversified, and no predictive factor has yet been identified or validated. New approaches looking for predictive proteins in the plasma are promising, helping to define the population that benefits from anti-VEGF treatment. New techniques such as NGS-based sequencing and whole-genome sequencing are becoming more widely used and affordable, and may help in the near future to detect novel biomarkers and guide treatment decisions. Although biomarker development during the past years has focused on targeted drugs, the most active substances in mCRC treatment remain cytotoxic chemotherapeutic drugs. To maximize the benefit/toxicity ratio, personalize treatment, and prolong OS, more efforts should be focused on biomarker development for 5-FU, oxaliplatin, and irinotecan.

Re-biopsies of tumor tissue and highly sensitive methods enabling clinicians to detect tumor changes during therapy in the blood will change concepts of treatment. The knowledge of resistance mechanisms and changes in tumor biology during therapy will help clinicians to make biologically rational decisions in the treatment sequence of mCRC.

REFERENCES

1. Siegel R, Ma J, Zou Z, et al. Cancer statistics, 2014. CA Cancer J Clin 2014;64(1):9–29.
2. Van Cutsem E, Kohne CH, Lang I, et al. Cetuximab plus irinotecan, fluorouracil, and leucovorin as first-line treatment for metastatic colorectal cancer: updated analysis of overall survival according to tumor KRAS and BRAF mutation status. J Clin Oncol 2011;29(15):2011–9.
3. Bennouna J, Sastre J, Arnold D, et al. Continuation of bevacizumab after first progression in metastatic colorectal cancer (ML18147): a randomised phase 3 trial. Lancet Oncol 2013;14(1):29–37.

4. O'Connell JB, Maggard MA, Ko CY. Colon cancer survival rates with the new American Joint Committee on Cancer sixth edition staging. J Natl Cancer Inst 2004;96(19):1420–5.

5. Tournigand C, Andre T, Achille E, et al. FOLFIRI followed by FOLFOX6 or the reverse sequence in advanced colorectal cancer: a randomized GERCOR study. J Clin Oncol 2004;22(2):229–37.

6. Saltz LB, Clarke S, Diaz-Rubio E, et al. Bevacizumab in combination with oxaliplatin-based chemotherapy as first-line therapy in metastatic colorectal cancer: a randomized phase III study. J Clin Oncol 2008;26(12):2013–9.

7. Cassidy J, Clarke S, Diaz-Rubio E, et al. XELOX vs FOLFOX-4 as first-line therapy for metastatic colorectal cancer: NO16966 updated results. Br J Cancer 2011; 105(1):58–64.

8. Hurwitz H, Fehrenbacher L, Novotny W, et al. Bevacizumab plus irinotecan, fluorouracil, and leucovorin for metastatic colorectal cancer. N Engl J Med 2004; 350(23):2335–42.

9. Bokemeyer C, Bondarenko I, Makhson A, et al. Fluorouracil, leucovorin, and oxaliplatin with and without cetuximab in the first-line treatment of metastatic colorectal cancer. J Clin Oncol 2009;27(5):663–71.

10. Douillard JY, Siena S, Cassidy J, et al. Randomized, phase III trial of panitumumab with infusional fluorouracil, leucovorin, and oxaliplatin (FOLFOX4) versus FOLFOX4 alone as first-line treatment in patients with previously untreated metastatic colorectal cancer: the PRIME study. J Clin Oncol 2010;28(31):4697–705.

11. Stintzing S, Lenz HJ. Protein kinase inhibitors in metastatic colorectal cancer. Let's pick patients, tumors, and kinase inhibitors to piece the puzzle together! Expert Opin Pharmacother 2013;14(16):2203–20.

12. Grothey A, Van Cutsem E, Sobrero A, et al. Regorafenib monotherapy for previously treated metastatic colorectal cancer (CORRECT): an international, multicentre, randomised, placebo-controlled, phase 3 trial. Lancet 2013;381(9863):303–12.

13. Joulain F, Proskorovsky I, Allegra C, et al. Mean overall survival gain with aflibercept plus FOLFIRI vs placebo plus FOLFIRI in patients with previously treated metastatic colorectal cancer. Br J Cancer 2013;109(7):1735–43.

14. Falcone A, Ricci S, Brunetti I, et al. Phase III trial of infusional fluorouracil, leucovorin, oxaliplatin, and irinotecan (FOLFOXIRI) compared with infusional fluorouracil, leucovorin, and irinotecan (FOLFIRI) as first-line treatment for metastatic colorectal cancer: the Gruppo Oncologico Nord Ovest. J Clin Oncol 2007; 25(13):1670–6.

15. Schmoll HJ, Van Cutsem E, Stein A, et al. ESMO Consensus Guidelines for management of patients with colon and rectal cancer. A personalized approach to clinical decision making. Ann Oncol 2012;23(10):2479–516.

16. Heinemann V, Stintzing S, Kirchner T, et al. Clinical relevance of EGFR- and KRAS-status in colorectal cancer patients treated with monoclonal antibodies directed against the EGFR. Cancer Treat Rev 2009;35(3):262–71.

17. Van Cutsem E, Peeters M, Siena S, et al. Open-label phase III trial of panitumumab plus best supportive care compared with best supportive care alone in patients with chemotherapy-refractory metastatic colorectal cancer. J Clin Oncol 2007;25(13):1658–64.

18. Jonker DJ, O'Callaghan CJ, Karapetis CS, et al. Cetuximab for the treatment of colorectal cancer. N Engl J Med 2007;357(20):2040–8.

19. Cunningham D, Humblet Y, Siena S, et al. Cetuximab monotherapy and cetuximab plus irinotecan in irinotecan-refractory metastatic colorectal cancer. N Engl J Med 2004;351(4):337–45.

20. Lievre A, Bachet JB, Le Corre D, et al. KRAS mutation status is predictive of response to cetuximab therapy in colorectal cancer. Cancer Res 2006;66(8): 3992–5.
21. Stintzing S, Fischer von Weikersthal L, Decker T, et al. FOLFIRI plus cetuximab versus FOLFIRI plus bevacizumab as first-line treatment for patients with metastatic colorectal cancer-subgroup analysis of patients with KRAS: mutated tumours in the randomised German AIO study KRK-0306. Ann Oncol 2012;23(7): 1693–9.
22. Chen CC, Er TK, Liu YY, et al. Computational analysis of KRAS mutations: implications for different effects on the KRAS p.G12D and p.G13D mutations. PLoS One 2013;8(2):e55793.
23. Irahara N, Baba Y, Nosho K, et al. NRAS mutations are rare in colorectal cancer. Diagn Mol Pathol 2010;19(3):157–63.
24. Douillard JY, Oliner KS, Siena S, et al. Panitumumab-FOLFOX4 treatment and RAS mutations in colorectal cancer. N Engl J Med 2013;369(11):1023–34.
25. Malumbres M, Barbacid M. RAS oncogenes: the first 30 years. Nat Rev Cancer 2003;3(6):459–65.
26. Tejpar S, Lenz HJ, Kohne CH, et al. Effect of KRAS and NRAS mutations on treatment outcomes in patients with metastatic colorectal cancer (mCRC) treated first-line with cetuximab plus FOLFOX4: New results from the OPUS study. J Clin Oncol 2014;32(Suppl 3) [abstract: LBA444].
27. Heinemann V, von Weikersthal LF, Decker T, et al. FOLFIRI plus cetuximab versus FOLFIRI plus bevacizumab as first-line treatment for patients with metastatic colorectal cancer (FIRE-3): a randomised, open-label, phase 3 trial. Lancet Oncol 2014;15(10):1065–75.
28. Brodowicz T, Vrbanec D, Kaczirek K, et al. FOLFOX4 plus cetuximab administered weekly or every two weeks in first-line treatment of patients with KRAS and NRAS wild-type (wt) metastatic colorectal cancer (mCRC). J Clin Oncol 2014;32(Suppl 3) [abstract: LBA391].
29. Schubbert S, Shannon K, Bollag G. Hyperactive Ras in developmental disorders and cancer. Nat Rev Cancer 2007;7(4):295–308.
30. Zuo Z, Chen SS, Chandra PK, et al. Application of COLD-PCR for improved detection of KRAS mutations in clinical samples. Mod Pathol 2009;22(8): 1023–31.
31. Anderson SM. Laboratory methods for KRAS mutation analysis. Expert Rev Mol Diagn 2011;11(6):635–42.
32. Janne PA, Borras AM, Kuang Y, et al. A rapid and sensitive enzymatic method for epidermal growth factor receptor mutation screening. Clin Cancer Res 2006;12(3 Pt 1):751–8.
33. Li M, Diehl F, Dressman D, et al. BEAMing up for detection and quantification of rare sequence variants. Nat Methods 2006;3(2):95–7.
34. Domagala P, Hybiak J, Sulzyc-Bielicka V, et al. KRAS mutation testing in colorectal cancer as an example of the pathologist's role in personalized targeted therapy: a practical approach. Pol J Pathol 2012;63(3):145–64.
35. Lee S, Brophy VH, Cao J, et al. Analytical performance of a PCR assay for the detection of KRAS mutations (codons 12/13 and 61) in formalin-fixed paraffin-embedded tissue samples of colorectal carcinoma. Virchows Arch 2012; 460(2):141–9.
36. Carotenuto P, Roma C, Rachiglio AM, et al. Detection of KRAS mutations in colorectal carcinoma patients with an integrated PCR/sequencing and real-time PCR approach. Pharmacogenomics 2010;11(8):1169–79.

37. Basso M, Strippoli A, Orlandi A, et al. KRAS mutational status affects oxaliplatin-based chemotherapy independently from basal mRNA ERCC-1 expression in metastatic colorectal cancer patients. Br J Cancer 2013;108(1):115–20.
38. Lin YL, Liau JY, Yu SC, et al. KRAS mutation is a predictor of oxaliplatin sensitivity in colon cancer cells. PLoS One 2012;7(11):e50701.
39. Schmiegel W, Reinacher-Schick A, Arnold D, et al. Capecitabine/irinotecan or capecitabine/oxaliplatin in combination with bevacizumab is effective and safe as first-line therapy for metastatic colorectal cancer: a randomized phase II study of the AIO colorectal study group. Ann Oncol 2013;24(6):1580–7.
40. Lin JS, Webber EM, Senger CA, et al. Systematic review of pharmacogenetic testing for predicting clinical benefit to anti-EGFR therapy in metastatic colorectal cancer. Am J Cancer Res 2011;1(5):650–62.
41. Sahin IH, Kazmi SM, Yorio JT, et al. Rare though not mutually exclusive: a report of three cases of concomitant KRAS and BRAF mutation and a review of the literature. J Cancer 2013;4(4):320–2.
42. Tol J, Nagtegaal ID, Punt CJ. BRAF mutation in metastatic colorectal cancer. N Engl J Med 2009;361(1):98–9.
43. Richman SD, Seymour MT, Chambers P, et al. KRAS and BRAF mutations in advanced colorectal cancer are associated with poor prognosis but do not preclude benefit from oxaliplatin or irinotecan: results from the MRC FOCUS trial. J Clin Oncol 2009;27(35):5931–7.
44. Price TJ, Hardingham JE, Lee CK, et al. Impact of KRAS and BRAF gene mutation status on outcomes from the phase III AGITG MAX trial of capecitabine alone or in combination with bevacizumab and mitomycin in advanced colorectal cancer. J Clin Oncol 2011;29(19):2675–82.
45. Loupakis F, Cremolini C, Salvatore L, et al. FOLFOXIRI plus bevacizumab as first-line treatment in BRAF mutant metastatic colorectal cancer. Eur J Cancer 2014; 50(1):57–63.
46. Shen Y, Wang J, Han X, et al. Effectors of epidermal growth factor receptor pathway: the genetic profiling of KRAS, BRAF, PIK3CA, NRAS mutations in colorectal cancer characteristics and personalized medicine. PLoS One 2013;8(12): e81628.
47. Seymour MT, Brown SR, Middleton G, et al. Panitumumab and irinotecan versus irinotecan alone for patients with KRAS wild-type, fluorouracil-resistant advanced colorectal cancer (PICCOLO): a prospectively stratified randomised trial. Lancet Oncol 2013;14(8):749–59.
48. Stintzing S, Lenz HJ. A small cog in a big wheel: PIK3CA mutations in colorectal cancer. J Natl Cancer Inst 2013;105(23):1775–6.
49. Janku F, Lee JJ, Tsimberidou AM, et al. PIK3CA mutations frequently coexist with RAS and BRAF mutations in patients with advanced cancers. PLoS One 2011; 6(7):e22769.
50. Liao X, Lochhead P, Nishihara R, et al. Aspirin use, tumor PIK3CA mutation, and colorectal-cancer survival. N Engl J Med 2012;367(17):1596–606.
51. Kothari N, Kim RD, Gibbs P, et al. Regular aspirin (ASA) use and survival in patients with PIK3CA-mutated metastatic colorectal cancer (CRC). J Clin Oncol 2014;32(Suppl 3) [abstract: 386].
52. De Roock W, De Vriendt V, Normanno N, et al. KRAS, BRAF, PIK3CA, and PTEN mutations: implications for targeted therapies in metastatic colorectal cancer. Lancet Oncol 2011;12(6):594–603.
53. Britten CD. PI3K and MEK inhibitor combinations: examining the evidence in selected tumor types. Cancer Chemother Pharmacol 2013;71(6):1395–409.

54. Yang ZY, Wu XY, Huang YF, et al. Promising biomarkers for predicting the outcomes of patients with KRAS wild-type metastatic colorectal cancer treated with anti-epidermal growth factor receptor monoclonal antibodies: a systematic review with meta-analysis. Int J Cancer 2013;133(8):1914–25.

55. Majek O, Gondos A, Jansen L, et al. Sex differences in colorectal cancer survival: population-based analysis of 164,996 colorectal cancer patients in Germany. PLoS One 2013;8(7):e68077.

56. Molinari F, Frattini M. Functions and regulation of the PTEN gene in colorectal cancer. Front Oncol 2013;3:326.

57. Sood A, McClain D, Maitra R, et al. PTEN gene expression and mutations in the PIK3CA gene as predictors of clinical benefit to anti-epidermal growth factor receptor antibody therapy in patients with KRAS wild-type metastatic colorectal cancer. Clin Colorectal Cancer 2012;11(2):143–50.

58. Danielsen SA, Lind GE, Bjornslett M, et al. Novel mutations of the suppressor gene PTEN in colorectal carcinomas stratified by microsatellite instability- and TP53 mutation-status. Hum Mutat 2008;29(11):E252–62.

59. Sartore-Bianchi A, Martini M, Molinari F, et al. PIK3CA mutations in colorectal cancer are associated with clinical resistance to EGFR-targeted monoclonal antibodies. Cancer Res 2009;69(5):1851–7.

60. Loupakis F, Pollina L, Stasi I, et al. PTEN expression and KRAS mutations on primary tumors and metastases in the prediction of benefit from cetuximab plus irinotecan for patients with metastatic colorectal cancer. J Clin Oncol 2009;27(16): 2622–9.

61. Tol J, Dijkstra JR, Klomp M, et al. Markers for EGFR pathway activation as predictor of outcome in metastatic colorectal cancer patients treated with or without cetuximab. Eur J Cancer 2010;46(11):1997–2009.

62. Khambata-Ford S, Garrett CR, Meropol NJ, et al. Expression of epiregulin and amphiregulin and K-ras mutation status predict disease control in metastatic colorectal cancer patients treated with cetuximab. J Clin Oncol 2007;25(22): 3230–7.

63. Jacobs B, De Roock W, Piessevaux H, et al. Amphiregulin and epiregulin mRNA expression in primary tumors predicts outcome in metastatic colorectal cancer treated with cetuximab. J Clin Oncol 2009;27(30):5068–74.

64. Jonker DJ, Karapetis CS, Harbison C, et al. Epiregulin gene expression as a biomarker of benefit from cetuximab in the treatment of advanced colorectal cancer. Br J Cancer 2014;110(3):648–55.

65. Stintzing S, Jung A, Kapaun C, et al. Amphiregulin and epiregulin expression predicts treatment efficacy in metastatic colorectal cancer (mCRC) patients treated with cetuximab plus CAPIRI or CAPOX: analysis of the German AIO CRC Group trial: KRK-0204. Ann Oncol 2011;22(Suppl 5):v10–8.

66. Lieu CH, Tran H, Jiang ZQ, et al. The association of alternate VEGF ligands with resistance to anti-VEGF therapy in metastatic colorectal cancer. PLoS One 2013; 8(10):e77117.

67. Vasudev NS, Reynolds AR. Anti-angiogenic therapy for cancer: current progress, unresolved questions and future directions. Angiogenesis 2014;17:471–94.

68. Formica V, Palmirotta R, Del Monte G, et al. Predictive value of VEGF gene polymorphisms for metastatic colorectal cancer patients receiving first-line treatment including fluorouracil, irinotecan, and bevacizumab. Int J Colorectal Dis 2011; 26(2):143–51.

69. Kopetz S, Hoff PM, Morris JS, et al. Phase II trial of infusional fluorouracil, irinotecan, and bevacizumab for metastatic colorectal cancer: efficacy and circulating

angiogenic biomarkers associated with therapeutic resistance. J Clin Oncol 2010;28(3):453–9.

70. Gianni L, Romieu GH, Lichinitser M, et al. AVEREL: a randomized phase III trial evaluating bevacizumab in combination with docetaxel and trastuzumab as first-line therapy for HER2-positive locally recurrent/metastatic breast cancer. J Clin Oncol 2013;31(14):1719–25.

71. Longley DB, Harkin DP, Johnston PG. 5-Fluorouracil: mechanisms of action and clinical strategies. Nat Rev Cancer 2003;3(5):330–8.

72. Walther A, Johnstone E, Swanton C, et al. Genetic prognostic and predictive markers in colorectal cancer. Nat Rev Cancer 2009;9(7):489–99.

73. Diasio RB, Johnson MR. The role of pharmacogenetics and pharmacogenomics in cancer chemotherapy with 5-fluorouracil. Pharmacology 2000;61(3):199–203.

74. Koopman M, Venderbosch S, van Tinteren H, et al. Predictive and prognostic markers for the outcome of chemotherapy in advanced colorectal cancer, a retrospective analysis of the phase III randomised CAIRO study. Eur J Cancer 2009; 45(11):1999–2006.

75. Vallbohmer D, Yang DY, Kuramochi H, et al. DPD is a molecular determinant of capecitabine efficacy in colorectal cancer. Int J Oncol 2007;31(2):413–8.

76. Teh LK, Hamzah S, Hashim H, et al. Potential of dihydropyrimidine dehydrogenase genotypes in personalizing 5-fluorouracil therapy among colorectal cancer patients. Ther Drug Monit 2013;35(5):624–30.

77. Popat S, Matakidou A, Houlston RS. Thymidylate synthase expression and prognosis in colorectal cancer: a systematic review and meta-analysis. J Clin Oncol 2004;22(3):529–36.

78. Pullarkat ST, Stoehlmacher J, Ghaderi V, et al. Thymidylate synthase gene polymorphism determines response and toxicity of 5-FU chemotherapy. Pharmacogenomics J 2001;1(1):65–70.

79. Kweekel DM, Gelderblom H, Guchelaar HJ. Pharmacology of oxaliplatin and the use of pharmacogenomics to individualize therapy. Cancer Treat Rev 2005;31(2): 90–105.

80. Grothey A, Goldberg RM. A review of oxaliplatin and its clinical use in colorectal cancer. Expert Opin Pharmacother 2004;5(10):2159–70.

81. Fischer von Weikersthal L, Schalhorn A, Stauch M, et al. Phase III trial of irinotecan plus infusional 5-fluorouracil/folinic acid versus irinotecan plus oxaliplatin as first-line treatment of advanced colorectal cancer. Eur J Cancer 2011;47(2):206–14.

82. Shirota Y, Stoehlmacher J, Brabender J, et al. ERCC1 and thymidylate synthase mRNA levels predict survival for colorectal cancer patients receiving combination oxaliplatin and fluorouracil chemotherapy. J Clin Oncol 2001;19(23):4298–304.

83. Ruzzo A, Graziano F, Loupakis F, et al. Pharmacogenetic profiling in patients with advanced colorectal cancer treated with first-line FOLFOX-4 chemotherapy. J Clin Oncol 2007;25(10):1247–54.

84. Baba H, Watanabe M, Okabe H, et al. Upregulation of ERCC1 and DPD expressions after oxaliplatin-based first-line chemotherapy for metastatic colorectal cancer. Br J Cancer 2012;107(12):1950–5.

85. Kanai M, Yoshioka A, Tanaka S, et al. Associations between glutathione S-transferase pi Ile105Val and glyoxylate aminotransferase Pro11Leu and Ile340Met polymorphisms and early-onset oxaliplatin-induced neuropathy. Cancer Epidemiol 2010;34(2):189–93.

86. Lamas MJ, Duran G, Balboa E, et al. Use of a comprehensive panel of biomarkers to predict response to a fluorouracil-oxaliplatin regimen in patients with metastatic colorectal cancer. Pharmacogenomics 2011;12(3):433–42.

87. Stoehlmacher J, Park DJ, Zhang W, et al. Association between glutathione S-transferase P1, T1, and M1 genetic polymorphism and survival of patients with metastatic colorectal cancer. J Natl Cancer Inst 2002;94(12):936–42.

88. Lamas MJ, Duran G, Balboa E, et al. The value of genetic polymorphisms to predict toxicity in metastatic colorectal patients with irinotecan-based regimens. Cancer Chemother Pharmacol 2012;69(6):1591–9.

89. Cunningham D, Pyrhonen S, James RD, et al. Randomised trial of irinotecan plus supportive care versus supportive care alone after fluorouracil failure for patients with metastatic colorectal cancer. Lancet 1998;352(9138):1413–8.

90. Douillard JY, Cunningham D, Roth AD, et al. Irinotecan combined with fluorouracil compared with fluorouracil alone as first-line treatment for metastatic colorectal cancer: a multicentre randomised trial. Lancet 2000;355(9209):1041–7.

91. Cecchin E, Innocenti F, D'Andrea M, et al. Predictive role of the UGT1A1, UGT1A7, and UGT1A9 genetic variants and their haplotypes on the outcome of metastatic colorectal cancer patients treated with fluorouracil, leucovorin, and irinotecan. J Clin Oncol 2009;27(15):2457–65.

92. Suenaga M, Fuse N, Yamaguchi T, et al. Pharmacokinetics, safety, and efficacy of FOLFIRI plus bevacizumab in Japanese colorectal cancer patients with UGT1A1 gene polymorphisms. J Clin Pharmacol 2014;54(5):495–502.

93. Braun MS, Richman SD, Quirke P, et al. Predictive biomarkers of chemotherapy efficacy in colorectal cancer: results from the UK MRC FOCUS trial. J Clin Oncol 2008;26(16):2690–8.

94. Nygard SB, Christensen IJ, Nielsen SL, et al. Assessment of the topoisomerase I gene copy number as a predictive biomarker of objective response to irinotecan in metastatic colorectal cancer. Scand J Gastroenterol 2014;49(1):84–91.

95. Moreira MC, Barbot C, Tachi N, et al. The gene mutated in ataxia-ocular apraxia 1 encodes the new HIT/Zn-finger protein aprataxin. Nat Genet 2001;29(2):189–93.

96. Dopeso H, Mateo-Lozano S, Elez E, et al. Aprataxin tumor levels predict response of colorectal cancer patients to irinotecan-based treatment. Clin Cancer Res 2010;16(8):2375–82.

Surgical Management of Hepatic Metastases of Colorectal Cancer

J. Joshua Smith, MD, PhD, Michael I. D'Angelica, MD*

KEYWORDS

- Colorectal cancer • Hepatic resection • Colorectal liver metastasis
- Hepatic arterial infusion

KEY POINTS

- Of the 136,000 patients diagnosed with colorectal cancer, 50% will develop metastases and most of these will be liver metastases, making colorectal liver metastases (CRLM) a significant public health problem.
- For the 20% of patients with resectable CRLM, hepatic resection is safe and effective, with an operative mortality of 1%, overall 5-year survival of 50% to 60%, and a 20% cure rate.
- Factors related to primary and metastatic tumors individually and in clinical risk-scoring schemes are the best prognostic factors; however, it is difficult to define patient groups with resectable, liver-limited CRLM that should be excluded from surgery.
- Systemic chemotherapy for metastatic colorectal cancer has improved; however, trials of adjuvant and/or neoadjuvant therapy around the time of hepatic resection have shown improvement in progression-free survival, but not overall survival.
- Conversion to complete resection with systemic and/or hepatic arterial infusion chemotherapy is a reasonable goal for patients with unresectable CRLM because outcomes are similar to those in patients with initially resectable disease.

INTRODUCTION, EPIDEMIOLOGY, AND NATURAL HISTORY

More than 90% of cancer-related mortality is due to metastatic disease and not from the primary tumors from which these arise.[1] Death from colorectal cancer is no different and, therefore, identification of optimal diagnostic, predictive, surgical, and perioperative modalities to prevent death from colorectal liver metastases is of paramount importance. Colorectal cancer is the third most common cancer in men and the

Conflicts of interest: None.
Department of Surgery, Memorial Sloan Kettering Cancer Center, 1275 York Avenue, New York, NY 10065, USA
* Corresponding author.
E-mail address: dangelim@mskcc.org

Hematol Oncol Clin N Am 29 (2015) 61–84
http://dx.doi.org/10.1016/j.hoc.2014.09.003
0889-8588/15/$ – see front matter © 2015 Elsevier Inc. All rights reserved.

second most common in women worldwide.[2] Approximately 96,000 patients will be diagnosed with colon cancer and 40,000 with rectal cancer in 2014[3]; unfortunately, 50,000 will die of their disease. Of the 136,000 patients diagnosed with colon and rectal cancer, 50% will develop metastases and a large proportion of these will be liver metastases.[4] Unresectable disease is the norm in these cases, but among the estimated 20% who are able to achieve complete resection there is an associated overall 5-year survival of 50% to 60%.[4] In fact, liver resection is the only treatment associated with long-term survival in patients with colorectal liver metastases (CRLM).[5,6] Furthermore, if patients are selected well, up to 20% are cured after hepatectomy for CRLM (**Fig. 1**).[7] This review describes the important aspects related to the surgical care of patients with CRLM.

Cattell performed what was probably the first hepatic resection for metastasis from the rectum in 1939, and reported that the patient was alive 12 months later. Early on, George Pack of Memorial Hospital in New York wrote that liver resection for CRLM was indicated when the primary tumor was controlled and a long interval had occurred between resection of the primary and discovery of the metastatic lesion. Interestingly Dr Quattlebaum, an early proponent of hepatic resection, proposed metastasectomy for "any and all" lesions unless the patient was deemed "incurable," a proposal that is still relevant, although incompletely defined, to the present day. Review of natural history data from the comprehensive monograph *Solid Liver Tumors* by Foster and Berman,[8] published in 1977, indicated that the mean survival for unresected CRLM ranged from 5 to 9 months in multiple series and that no survivors were noted at 5 years.[8] In a series of more than 1000 patients reported in 1990, median survival was 6.9 months for unresectable CRLM and 14.9 months for resectable disease that was not resected. However, if disease was resected with negative margins, the median survival was 30 months with a 38% 5-year survival.[9] It has become clear that without surgical management, median survival is measured in months and 5-year survival is rare. In the modern era, patients with resected CRLM now have an associated 5-year overall survival (OS) of 50% to 60% and a long-term cure rate of approximately 20% (**Table 1**).[10,11] Systemic chemotherapy for metastatic colorectal

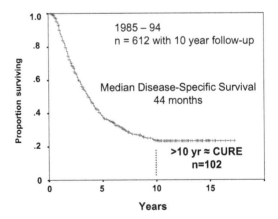

Fig. 1. Resection of colorectal liver metastases (CRLM) is safe and curative. Displayed is the 10-year follow-up on patients who underwent resection of CRLM from 1985 to 1994 at Memorial Sloan Kettering. There were 102 actual 10-year survivors, and 97% of the 102 were disease free at the last follow-up. (*Adapted from* Tomlinson JS, De Jarnagin WR, Matteo RP, et al. Actual 10-year survival after resection of colorectal liver metastases defines cure. J Clin Oncol 2007;25:4575–80; with permission.)

Table 1
Rationale for surgery and outcomes: selected series of studies and associated mortality and survival for CRLM demonstrating the trends over the last 30 years

Authors,[Ref.] Year	N	Mortality (%)	5-Year Survival (%)	10-Year Survival (%)
Hughes et al,[110] 1986	607	n/a	33	n/a
Scheele et al,[111] 1991	219	6	39	n/a
Gayowski et al,[112] 1994	204	0	32	n/a
Scheele et al,[62] 1995	469	4	39	20
Nordlinger et al,[113] 1996	1568	2	28	n/a
Jamison et al,[114] 1997	280	4	27	20
Fong et al,[5] 1999	1001	3	37	n/a
Choti et al,[10] 2002	226	1	40	n/a
Abdulla et al,[115] 2004	190	n/a	58	n/a
House et al,[45] 2010	1600			8-year
Era 1: 1985–1998	Era 1: 1037	Era 1: 2.5	Era 1: 37	Era 1: 26
Era 2: 1999–2004	Era 2: 563	Era 2: 1	Era 2: 51	Era 2: 37

Abbreviation: n/a, no data available.

cancer has improved over the last 2 decades. Although response rates typically exceed 50% and median survival in most trials approximates 2 years, 5-year survival is uncommon and long-term cure is exceedingly rare.[12]

Early reports on hepatic resection for CRLM were limited by small numbers, retrospective analyses, and susceptibility to selection bias. While 5-year survival was rare in patients who did not undergo surgery, it was possible that extreme selection of cases for resection resulted in higher percentages simply by altering the denominator. Silen[13] penned this opinion eloquently in 1989. Although the long-term survival in patients who undergo surgery for CRLM could theoretically be a result of patient selection, comparison between series of chemotherapy and surgery over the last 4 decades showed that the results were so dramatically different that it became difficult to argue against a role for surgery or to have sufficient equipoise for a randomized trial. The argument for hepatic resection is further strengthened by the fact that patients are cured by surgery at a rate similar to that of some primary nonmetastatic malignancies.

WORKUP AND STAGING

In the modern era, most CRLM are asymptomatic and are typically diagnosed with imaging studies either at diagnosis or during follow-up after treatment of the primary tumor.[4] For the purposes of detection and surveillance, the National Comprehensive Cancer Network (NCCN) guidelines recommend computed tomography (CT) scans to monitor for recurrence after resection of primary colorectal cancer, and additionally as a means of monitoring response and disease status in CRLM patients undergoing treatment.[14] Imaging to assess for the presence of metastatic disease at the time of primary tumor diagnosis is indicated given the multiple treatment options available for patients with CRLM. At the time of diagnosis of CRLM a baseline carcinoembryonic antigen (CEA) is helpful as a means of monitoring treatment response and/or recurrence. In those cases where metachronous CRLM is found, a colonoscopy within a year of the diagnosis is considered standard. For the patient found to have liver metastasis, staging consists of high-quality cross-sectional imaging of the chest, abdomen, and pelvis. In the case of an intact asymptomatic primary tumor, there is no urgency to resect the primary before addressing the metastasis.[15] Ultrasonography, MRI, and ^{18}F-fluorodeoxyglucose PET/CT are options for imaging, but the current standard is high-quality multiphasic cross-sectional imaging of the chest, abdomen, and pelvis. Chest imaging is typically obtained with CT, and imaging of the abdomen and pelvis can be obtained with CT and/or MRI. CRLM lesions on CT are hypovascular and are usually visualized as hypodense lesions on the portovenous phase. MRI can be a useful adjunct for liver-specific disease to better characterize subtle disease findings, and lesion characterization when not clear on CT. MRI can be particularly helpful in a steatotic liver or for disappearing metastases after chemotherapy exposure.[16]

Until recently, controversy existed regarding the utility of PET scanning over standard cross-sectional imaging in terms of staging patients with CRLM. In an early study of 40 patients with potentially resectable disease, findings on PET altered management of resection in 23% of the patients and influenced clinical decision making in 40% of patients.[17] Surgery was avoided in 5 cases of extrahepatic metastatic disease, and in 3 cases PET findings led to biopsies proving unresectable liver disease. A French study published in 2005 evaluated the cost-effectiveness of PET in the management of metachronous CRLM.[18] The study found that PET/CT was more cost-effective than CT alone, and that 6% of patients could avoid an unnecessary laparotomy. Although these results are intriguing, this model was based on retrospective data that were not validated. Recently, a randomized trial of PET/CT versus CT in patients with potentially resectable CRLM has been published.[19] The use of PET/CT did not result in significant changes in surgical management, and there was no difference in resectability or long-term outcomes between the 2 groups. This trial provides definitive evidence that the routine use of PET does not significantly affect outcomes among patients with potentially resectable CRLM.[19] The most recent NCCN guidelines for localized colon cancer do not recommend routine PET/CT for surveillance[20] or for monitoring therapeutic progress for metastatic colorectal cancer.[14] The authors believe that PET can be helpful in relatively uncommon selected situations where there are equivocal findings on CT or MRI that could significantly alter treatment.

RESECTABILITY: DEFINITIONS AND APPROACHES

The definition of resectability revolves around the technical aspects of achieving an R0 margin while sparing a sufficient remnant liver in addition to tumor biology, extent of disease, and risk of recurrence. The surgeon must consider the patient's ability to undergo the significant physiologic stress of a major operation and balance this against the likelihood of achieving an oncologic survival advantage. One should not confuse the ability to remove all CRLM with the underlying tumor biology that will determine outcome. Numerous techniques including parenchymal-sparing resections, intraoperative ablation, portal vein embolization, and 2-stage resections have improved our ability to safely remove larger burdens of disease while leaving a sufficient future liver remnant.[21] Although resectability can easily be defined in terms of technical ability to remove tumors, the authors consider that this is not a complete definition. Technical resectability (eg, ability to remove all the tumors) should be defined separately from biological resectability (eg, ability to achieve long-term survival and/or cure).

The presence of 4 or more metastases was a contraindication to hepatectomy in the past, owing to the very poor reported 5-year survival rates.[22] However, these studies were promulgated in times of inadequate staging, crude imaging, and ineffective chemotherapy.[23] Cady and colleagues[24] reported in 1992 a series of 129 patients who underwent resection for CRLM, and recommended that patients with more than 4 metastatic nodules not undergo attempted resection because of poor survival.

More recently, multiple groups have shown that long-term survival is possible in patients undergoing resection of 4 or more CRLM (23%–51% 5-year survival).[25–28] The limit on the number of metastatic lesions is still unclear, but one group reported that more than 8 metastatic lesions portends a particularly poor outcome.[28] These reports on patients with 4 or more metastases also report very high recurrence rates, although cure is typically documented in approximately 5% to 10% of patients. One must consider the selection bias in these studies as a limiting factor, in addition to weighing the benefits of surgery in a fair manner knowing that hepatectomy may provide long-term survival without actually rendering a cure.

It is now well accepted that positive margins are associated with worse outcomes, but it is not always possible to predict the pathologic margin status preoperatively. Although there is some disagreement, most series show that a positive margin is associated with poor outcome and uncommon long-term survival.[22,29] It should be noted that poor outcomes after a positive margin are not simply due to local recurrence at the margin. It is likely that this margin is a surrogate for particularly bad tumor biology. Most series indicate that negative margins, regardless of width, are associated with favorable outcomes.[30] However, work by the authors' group demonstrated that the width of the margin (>10 mm) was independently associated with outcome but that negative but close margins were still associated with favorable long-term survival.[31] A predicted close margin should not preclude hepatic resection, as it is impossible to predict margin positivity and patients with negative but close margins still have a significant chance of cure and long-term survival. Technique of hepatic resection may affect margin status and outcome. Scheele and colleagues[9] demonstrated that nonanatomic resection was associated with worse outcomes. DeMatteo and colleagues[32] studied 267 CRLM patients, and determined that segmentectomy was associated with wider margins and improved survival in comparison with wedge resections. The goal of surgery should be to obtain an R0 resection, and although nonanatomic wedge resections are sometimes sufficient, wider segmental resections probably provide a better chance of surgical success.

Another difficult consideration in terms of resectability is the presence of limited and resectable extrahepatic disease (EHD). Historically the presence of EHD was a contraindication because of its associated poor survival.[33] More modern series have demonstrated better long-term survival in patients with limited EHD.[34,35] However, even in these highly selected patients the recurrence rates are high and cure is rare. Therefore, surgical treatment should be used sparingly in these patients as a general rule, but in highly selected patients; especially those who have undergone and responded to systemic chemotherapy, surgery should be considered. The role of surgery in patients with EHD is discussed later in further detail.

In summary, patients with less than 4 metastases, no EHD, and tumors amenable to an R0 resection should undergo resection both for the obvious associated survival advantage and the potential for cure. Patients with 4 or more metastases, resectable EHD, and/or the likelihood of close margins have a significantly lower chance of cure but do have an associated better survival rate than chemotherapy alone. These high-risk patients must be carefully selected for operation and counseled about the high risk of recurrence, the need for careful surveillance, and the likelihood of reintervention with chemotherapy or surgery.

Historically resectability at the time of laparotomy was a significant issue, with many patients being found to have additional disease precluding resection. The rate of unresectable disease at laparotomy has previously been reported at 15% to 70%.[36,37] Recently the authors' group sought to analyze the rate of operative resectability in a modern cohort of 455 CLM patients.[38] Among these 455 patients, only 35 (7.7%)

were found to be unresectable at surgery. The reasons for unresectability were extensive liver-only disease (n = 15), EHD (n = 17), marked hepatic toxicity (n = 1), and extensive adhesions precluding safe conduct of the operation (n = 2). Of note, 45 patients were found to have EHD and 27 of these still underwent resection. This markedly improved rate of operative resectability reflects better preoperative imaging and staging in addition to the expansion of resectability criteria to include patients with limited EHD. The only factor associated with unresectable disease was a prior history of EHD. Diagnostic laparoscopy was used sparingly in this cohort, and among the 55 patients who underwent laparoscopy only 4 patients were found to be unresectable. Therefore, diagnostic laparoscopy has a low yield and should only be used for specific imaging findings that would preclude resection if found to be disease at surgery. Overall, the rate of operative resectability is high, and small minorities of patients undergo nontherapeutic laparotomy.

A significant operative hurdle exists among patients with synchronous resectable liver metastases with an intact primary tumor. Synchronous liver metastases are common, occurring in 25% of patients with colorectal cancer. Three surgical approaches can be taken for these patients.[39] A simultaneous approach combines the liver and colorectal operation into one operation. A staged approach with separate operations for the colorectal tumor and the liver was historically favored, and typically addressed the colorectal tumor first for fear of obstruction or bleeding. A more recent description of this staged approach involves liver resection first. Candidates for a liver-first approach need to have asymptomatic primaries and often have CRLM that require a major hepatectomy. A liver-first approach has also been used in patients with rectal primaries to allow for time to treat the rectal tumor with preoperative chemoradiation. Several retrospective comparisons of the 3 approaches have been published. Most show no significant differences in outcome, and some favor the simultaneous approach in terms of improved postoperative morbidity and decreased length of stay. These studies, however, are significantly biased in that the staged resections more often are in patients requiring a major hepatectomy and/or a complex rectal operation. Some studies have reported that major hepatectomy is associated with high mortality with the simultaneous approach[40]; however, most studies show that major hepatic resections can be safely carried out with a concomitant colorectal resection.[40,41] In the management of the patient with synchronous CRLM, early involvement of a hepatic surgeon is critical for treatment planning and success. In general, the authors advocate a simultaneous approach[39]; however, the controversy lies in those patients who may require an extensive rectal resection and a major hepatectomy, and it is certainly reasonable to consider a staged approach in such patients.

PROGNOSTIC FACTORS

Only decades ago, prognosis was uniformly poor for patients with unresected CRLM. Approximately 70% of patients with unresected CRLM died within 1 year, and survival beyond 5 years was rare.[42,43] Looking broadly across the CRLM population in 2 large academic centers in the United States encompassing 2470 patients, Kopetz and colleagues[44] demonstrated no significant difference in median OS for those diagnosed between 1990 and 1997, whereas significant improvements were noted in the groups diagnosed between 1998 and 2000 (18 months) and from 2004 to 2006 (29.2 months). The investigators attributed these improved survival rates to the more frequent adoption of hepatic resection and improved chemotherapeutic options. In a recent study from the authors' group, differences in long-term outcomes were analyzed in 1600 patients who underwent resection of CRLM in 2 eras: 1985 to 1998 (n = 1037) and 1999 to 2004 (n = 563).[45] One important finding of this study was that operative mortality was significantly less in the modern era (1% vs 2.5%). Furthermore, despite relatively worse biological characteristics, median survival improved from 43 to 64 months. These data suggest that the survival rate for CRLM has improved over time, which likely reflects better patient selection, appropriate chemotherapeutic choices, and better operative management.

Over the last few decades many retrospective case series of patients undergoing hepatic resection for CRLM have reported on individual predictors of survival. The most common predictors of shorter survival were increasing size and number of tumors, shorter disease-free interval, node-positive primary tumor, positive margins, and the presence of EHD. These individual prognostic factors, however, vary from study to study in their association with outcomes, and have not been consistent across studies. In 1999, in an attempt to improve prognostication, a Clinical Risk Score (CRS) that predicts survival after hepatic resection for CRLM was developed by Fong and colleagues[5] using data from 1001 patients treated from 1985 to 1998 at Memorial Sloan Kettering Cancer Center (MSKCC). The 5 preoperative factors found to be independent predictors of poor outcomes were node-positive primary, disease-free interval less than 12 months, more than 1 tumor, largest tumor greater than 5 cm, and CEA greater than 200 ng/mL. The CRS is constructed by adding a point for each of the 5 factors, and this score correlated well with outcomes. Interestingly neither the CRS nor other individual factors precluded the possibility of cure. In the authors' published series, the only factor that did preclude cure was a positive margin.[7] Whereas the CRS remains a useful prognostic tool in the authors' hands, it has not translated well across all institutions. Specifically, Zakaria and colleagues[46] showed that the CRS had limited prognostic value in their cohort from the Mayo Clinic. Furthermore, these prognostic factors, including the CRS, do not necessarily exclude patients from resection given the possibility of long-term survival, even with poor prognostic factors limiting the clinical applicability.

Other prognostic tools have been developed to help predict outcome among patients undergoing hepatic resection for CRLM. Using 1477 CRLM patients from 1986 to 1999, a nomogram was developed incorporating several of the CRS elements, resection characteristics, and colon or rectal origin to predict 96-month disease-specific survival. Importantly this nomogram was validated in an external data set.[47] In other work, a Japanese group developed both a preoperative and postoperative nomogram in 578 CRLM patients to predict 5-year disease-specific survival (DSS) using 6 clinical variables.[48] Nomograms are potentially useful tools because they are dynamic, can adapt readily to clinical, pathologic, and genomic information, and provide a more precise assessment of individual risk.[49] However, nomograms are susceptible to selection bias, can vary by institution, and often are not useful in making clinical decisions. The biggest issue among nomograms and risk-scoring systems is that it is often difficult to define groups with such a poor outcome that surgery is not advised, limiting their clinical applicability. The authors' group has recently used the CRS and gene-expression data to better determine risk in patients with CRLM. Tumor tissue from 96 patients who underwent R0 resection were used to develop a gene-expression profile associated with outcomes. A Molecular Risk Score (MRS) was constructed and then evaluated in a test set.[50] The MRS predicted survival independently of the CRS and, when combined with the CRS, allowed powerful prediction of outcomes (**Fig. 2**). It remains to be seen whether the MRS can be validated in an external data set to better delineate risk allocation in CRLM patients.

Given the difficulty with predicting outcome with clinical factors alone, investigators have explored the prognostic role of immunomodulatory and inflammatory markers. In

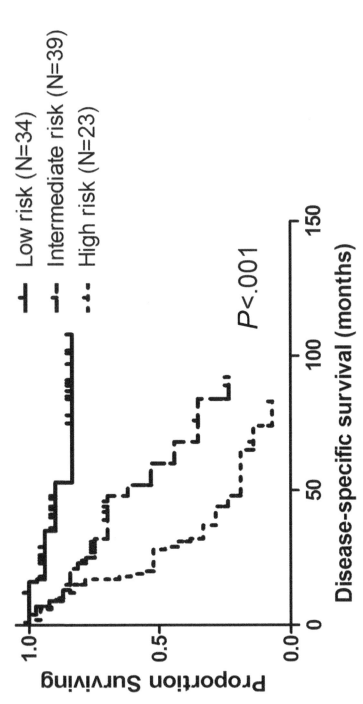

Fig. 2. Risk stratification by combination of Clinical Risk Score (CRS) and Molecular Risk Score (MRS) for disease-specific survival (DSS). Genes identified in liver metastases of 96 patients who underwent and R0 liver resection were analyzed by gene-expression analysis, and an MRS was constructed by Cox regression and evaluated in both training and test sets. Kaplan-Meier estimates of DSS are shown for patients with metastatic colorectal cancer in the high-, intermediate-, and very low-risk groups across both the training (n = 60) and test set (n = 36). These data demonstrate the high prognostic value of the MRS expression profile in patients with completely resected hepatic metastases from colorectal cancer. (*Adapted from* Ito H, Mo Q, Qin LX, et al. Gene expression profiles accurately predict outcome following liver resection in patients with metastatic colorectal cancer. PLoS One 2013;8(12):e81680.)

a study of 170 patients undergoing resection for CRLM, an elevated serum C-reactive protein (a marker of systemic inflammation) level was associated with worse disease-free survival (DFS) (19 vs 43 months).[51] In a separate study, an elevated serum neutrophil-to-lymphocyte ratio was associated with worse survival.[52] Other studies have addressed tumor immune infiltrates of the CRLM. One study of 162 CRLM patients with longer survival times demonstrated tumors with a higher proportion of CD8[+] T cells versus CD4[+] T cells, and the combination of these 2 provided the best prediction of long-term good outcomes.[53] An immunohistochemical analysis of chemokine receptors and ligands in CRLM implicated CXCR4 expression in tumors as potentially worthy of future study as a prognostic marker.[54] These data indicate that the complex signaling and fine adaptations by the immune system/stroma and the epithelial cells during the formation and maintenance of a metastatic lesion in the liver may play an important role in terms of survival and recurrence end points.

Although not helpful in the preoperative setting, the timing and pattern of recurrence after hepatectomy for CRLM have been found to be relevant prognostic factors. Among a group of 637 resected CRLM patients, 62% recurred and the initial patterns were liver only (31%), lung only (27%), multiple sites (30%), and other single sites (12%). Recurrence pattern, time to recurrence, and resection of recurrence all independently correlated with survival.[23] Additional research has shown that early postoperative recurrence within 1 year of hepatic resection is the single most important variable in terms of estimating DSS in conditional models of prediction and outcome.[55] These data demonstrate that recurrence after hepatectomy occurs in definable patterns, and time and pattern of recurrence are probably important predictors of outcome.

OPERATIVE OUTCOMES: FACTORS AFFECTING MORBIDITY AND MORTALITY

Hepatic resection historically has been viewed as a high-risk operation. Initial reports demonstrated that mortality was high,[8] and early reviews demonstrated an operative mortality ranging from 8% to 40% with an average operative mortality of 21%.[56] Fortunately, the safety of liver resection for malignancy has improved dramatically over the last few decades. A recent review of the National Surgical Quality Improvement Program (NSQIP) on 2313 patients indicated a post-hepatectomy 30-day mortality of 2.5% and 30-day major morbidity of 20% nationally.[57] Morbidity and mortality rates parallel the extent of resection. For example, in the NSQIP study 30-day mortality rates for a partial, left, right, and extended hepatectomy were 1.8%, 0.9%, 3.7%, and 5.2%, respectively. Factors found to be associated with increased morbidity were elevated American Society of Anesthesiologists score, smoking, elevated alkaline phosphatase, hypoalbuminemia, elevated partial thromboplastin time, intraoperative transfusion, postoperative transfusion, and operative time. Overall mortality for hepatic resection for CRLM is currently less than 1% at most referral or tertiary centers; a true testament to improved patient selection and operative technique.[58]

The importance of morbidity may also lie in its potential effects on long-term oncologic outcomes. In a study of 1067 patients undergoing liver resection for CRLM, postoperative morbidity was independently associated with oncologic outcomes in multivariate analysis.[59] DSS and DFS for patients with complications was 41% and 25%, whereas for those patients who did not have a complication their DSS and DFS were significantly higher at 48% and 33%, respectively. A recent meta-analysis by Matsuda and colleagues[60] analyzing 4 studies involving 2280 CRLM patients looked specifically at the influence of postoperative complications on DFS and OS. For both DFS and OS, their data indicate postoperative complications have a significant negative impact on both recurrence and survival. The reasons for worse outcomes after a postoperative complication are complex, but may be associated with a delay in adjuvant therapy administration and/or the inflammatory/immunosuppressive state that may promote cancer progression. These data serve as a stark reminder that hepatic resection for CRLM requires meticulous attention in the operating room and cautious perioperative management with an eye toward minimization of postoperative complications.

Patients with bilobar metastases pose a significant difficulty, as there are many potential methods of resecting disease. In a recent study, 440 CRLM patients with bilobar disease were retrospectively analyzed to evaluate morbidity, mortality, and evolution of technical approaches over time. During the period of this study (1992–2003) the techniques of addressing bilateral disease changed significantly over time, with a move away from extended or hemi-hepatectomies and a move toward multiple, smaller resections. Overall there was a 29% rate of major complications and 5% 90-day mortality.[61] Over the course of 10 years the rate of major hepatectomy decreased from 90% to 75% while the rate of wedge resection increased from 15% to nearly 40%. Concurrent with evolution toward a parenchymal-sparing approach, the 90-day mortality decreased from 6.3% to 1.2%. Of importance, DSS and DFS were no different over the time period. These data demonstrate that parenchymal-sparing surgery in the setting of bilateral CRLM is associated with decreased mortality and does not affect oncologic outcomes.

Perioperative blood transfusions have been purported to affect perioperative morbidity and long-term oncologic outcomes in many cancer types. Because of a historically high operative blood loss, many centers used transfusion routinely in the past for hepatic surgery.[62–66] However, today blood transfusions have become much less common.[67] In an analysis of 1351 CRLM patients undergoing resection at MSKCC from 1986 to 2001, transfusion was associated with significantly worse perioperative morbidity. Nontransfused patients had significantly fewer complications and shorter lengths of stay even if the comparison group only included patients receiving 1 or 2 units of blood. Blood transfusion of any kind did not remain as a significant predictor of long-term survival when entered into a multivariate model including tumor-related variables. These data indicate that transfusion-associated adverse effects are most relevant in the perioperative period and, if possible, transfusions should be avoided.

Many strategies have been put forth to reduce blood transfusions. Intraoperative blood loss has been reduced by a better understanding of hepatic anatomy, experience at high-volume centers, and improved instrumentation. Perhaps the most important step in decreasing blood loss was the appreciation that most blood loss came from hepatic veins and that maintenance of low central venous pressure during hepatic transection can significantly decrease blood loss.[21] This strategy requires preoperative management planning by anesthesia to limit pretransection fluid volume and to treat central venous pressure (CVP) actively if needed. The seminal article by Melendez and colleagues[68] showed dramatic reductions in blood loss, morbidity, and mortality with low CVP, and in parallel demonstrated no impact on perioperative renal function. Another potential way to reduce blood transfusion is acute normovolemic hemodilution (ANH). ANH is a blood-conservation technique whereby whole blood is removed intraoperatively before incision to a predetermined serum hemoglobin level, with maintenance of isovolemia using crystalloid or colloid replacement.[69] Blood withdrawn is reinfused during the procedure if needed or after the completion of the operation. In a recent randomized trial ANH was associated with fewer blood transfusions, and the effect was particularly pronounced in patients who had a blood loss of greater than 800 mL.[69]

EXTRAHEPATIC DISEASE: RESECTABILITY, OUTCOMES, AND SITE-SPECIFIC FACTORS

The most consistent contraindication to hepatic resection for CRLM has been the presence of EHD.[22] In an early report, Adson and colleagues[70] indicated that EHD precluded 5-year survival. An extensive review by Blumgart and Fong[33] in 1995 stated "at present, extrahepatic disease and inability to resect all hepatic disease are the only absolute contraindications to resection." The role of surgery for patients with EHD has been questioned more recently because older studies were based on small cohorts, in an era of ineffective chemotherapy and poor imaging. More modern studies have suggested that there is a role for resection of CRLM in highly selected patients with limited and resectable EHD. Elias and colleagues[34] reviewed outcomes of 224 CRLM patients without EHD and compared them with 84 patients with EHD, and found that the patients without EHD had a significantly better outcomes (28% vs 34% 5-year survival, $P = .04$). The investigators evaluated OS for each group when looking at the number of liver-only metastases versus the total number of metastases for each group, and proposed that prognostication based on total number of metastases may be more reliable. This study has been criticized for methodological flaws; however, as a result of the long-term survival it provided data to suggest that EHD, when resectable, was no longer an absolute contraindication to resection.

The authors analyzed 127 CRLM patients at MSKCC with radiographically or intraoperatively detected EHD.[35] These 127 patients constituted 8.5% of the 1359 hepatic resections for CRLM from 1992 to 2007. Patients without EHD had better survival than those with EHD (5-year survival 26% vs 49%, $P<.001$). Among the patients with EHD, survival was best for patients with lung, ovarian and limited peritoneal disease and worst for patients with portal lymph node involvement. Most importantly, 95% of the patients who underwent complete resection ultimately recurred, and the median time to recurrence was 9 months. In summary, these data indicate that long-term survival can be realized in this these highly selected patients with limited and resectable EHD, but cure is rare.

Initial experience by the Thoracic Surgery Group at MSKCC demonstrated that survival rates for resection of colorectal pulmonary metastases were 44% (5-year) and 30% (10-year) in an analysis of 144 patients, demonstrating that resection of colorectal lung metastases is associated with a long-term survival.[71] On the other hand, review of 131 patients undergoing liver and lung resection for CRLM between 1981 and 2000 demonstrated that resection of pulmonary metastases is feasible, and that longer survival was associated with patients younger than 55 years, with solitary liver metastasis, and a disease-free interval greater than 1 year, whereas nodal status, CEA, adjuvant chemotherapy, or characteristics of the pulmonary metastases was not.[72] The 5-year survival rate for a disease-free interval greater than 12 months was 64%, compared with 23% when the disease-free interval was less than 12 months. In regard to subcentimeter pulmonary nodules found on staging workup for resectable CRLM, recent analysis of 160 CRLM patients from the authors' group indicates that even though one-third of these will be metastatic disease, 3-year DSS is not affected, and these patients should still undergo hepatectomy if indicated.[73]

ADJUVANT AND NEOADJUVANT CHEMOTHERAPY

Systemic chemotherapy has dramatically improved for patients with unresectable metastatic colorectal cancer.[12] With these improvements it was hoped that systemic chemotherapy would improve outcomes as with adjuvant therapy in patients undergoing complete resection of CRLM. Unfortunately, randomized trials have not shown a dramatic improvement in outcomes with modern systemic therapy administered before and/or after hepatic resection.

In an analysis of pooled data on 302 patients from 2 prospective randomized trials comparing hepatic resection alone with hepatic resection combined with adjuvant 5-fluorouracil (5-FU)/leucovorin (LV), there was no demonstrable improvement in OS. Adjuvant 5-FU/LV was associated with a trend toward an improved progression-free survival (PFS) (median 28 vs 19 months, $P = .06$), but there was no statistically significant impact on OS (median 62 vs 47 months, $P = .1$). Ychou and colleagues demonstrated in a prospective randomized trial of 306 patients who underwent an R0 metastasectomy randomized to 5-FU/LV compared with FOLFIRI (leucovorin/5-FU/irinotecan) from 2001 to 2006 that there was no significant improvement in OS or PFS, indicating that irinotecan lacks activity in this postresection setting. The European Organization for Research and Treatment of Cancer (EORTC) 40983 trial by Nordlinger and colleagues[74] in 2008 randomized 364 patients with fewer than 4 metastases to perioperative (pre- and postoperative) FOLFOX (leucovorin/5-FU/oxaliplatin) versus surgery alone. There was a statistical trend toward a significant 7% absolute improvement in PFS at 3 years ($P = .06$). Of note, the improved PFS is seen at the initial time point in the trial. The reason for this is unclear, but may be related to early progression in the surgery-alone group. A recent update with long-term follow-up did not demonstrate an improved OS with perioperative FOLFOX, although the trial was not specifically powered to detect small differences in OS. In addition, recent work on the use of cetuximab plus chemotherapy in patients with resectable CRLM indicated that KRAS exon 2 wild-type patients had worse DFS ($P = .03$) and trended toward worse OS ($P = .16$), demonstrating no benefit for the addition of cetuximab in this setting.[75] In sum, these trials show small and often insignificant improvements in PFS and, although underpowered, have not shown an improvement in OS (**Table 2**).

After resection of CRLM the most common site of recurrence is the liver, which is involved in approximately half of the cases of recurrence; therefore, the authors' group has studied the use of adjuvant hepatic arterial infusion pumps (HAIP) with floxuridine (FUDR).[76] A randomized controlled trial of adjuvant HAIP with FUDR combined with systemic 5-FU/LV compared with systemic 5-FU/LV alone showed better hepatic relapse-free survival and OS in the hepatic arterial infusion (HAI) group.[77,78] Median OS for HAI patients was 72 months in comparison with 59 months ($P = .03$). More impressively, median hepatic PFS was 90% in comparison with 60% at 2 years ($P<.001$). An updated analysis of this trial with long-term follow-up showed a trend toward better long-term OS in the HAI group (median 68.4 vs 58.8 months) and a

Table 2
Randomized prospective trials of perioperative chemotherapy in CRLM over the past 5 years showing no significant improvement in survival

Authors,[Ref.] Year	Comparison	N	PFS	OS
Mitry et al,[86] 2008	5-FU vs observation	302	Trend ($P = .058$)	No ($P = .095$)
Ychou et al,[87] 2009	FOLFIRI vs 5-FU	306	No ($P = .44$)	No ($P = .69$)
Nordlinger et al,[74] 2013	FOLFOX4 vs observation	364	Trend ($P = .068$)	No ($P = .34$)
Primrose et al,[75] 2014	FOLFOX vs FOLFOX plus cetuximab	257	$P = .03$ (CTX plus cetuximab did worse)	No ($P = .16$)

Abbreviations: 5-FU, 5-fluorouracil; CTX, cyclophosphamide; FOLFIRI, leucovorin/5-FU/irinotecan; FOLFOX, leucovorin/5-FU/oxaliplatin; OS, overall survival; PFS, progression-free survival.

significantly longer PFS in the HAIP+systemic group versus systemic alone[78] (median 31.3 vs 17.2 months). Although this initial trial showed improved outcomes over adjuvant 5-FU/LV, the relevance of this finding in the current era of improved systemic therapy has been questioned. However, adjuvant HAI treatment has also evolved and is now routinely combined with modern systemic chemotherapy.[21,79] Outcomes in patients receiving modern regimens of chemotherapy with or without HAI-FUDR have been recently compared in a retrospective study by House and colleagues[80] in 250 patients undergoing CRLM resection. At a median follow-up of 43 months, adjuvant HAI-FUDR was associated with a significantly better OS and hepatic recurrence-free survival. This study supports the concept that HAI-FUDR and modern systemic therapy may be a more effective adjuvant regimen than modern systemic chemotherapy alone, and probably justifies a randomized trial. Kemeny and colleagues[81] investigated the addition of bevacizumab to adjuvant HAI plus systemic therapy after liver resection in a randomized phase II study. This study was terminated early because of significantly worse biliary toxicity in the bevacizumab arm. The addition of bevacizumab to adjuvant HAI plus systemic chemotherapy did not improve outcomes; however, 4-year survival was impressive (85% and 81% in each group, $P = .5$). Complications can occur with HAIP, such as biliary toxicity (unresectable [2%] vs resected [5%]),[82] but are typically managed with dose reduction and steroids.

The rationale for neoadjuvant therapy for resectable CRLM is based on the idea that early eradication of microscopic metastatic disease is beneficial, and that this therapy can be used to identify active (or inactive) chemotherapy and help select patients for surgery. Some of the data to support this idea come from a retrospective study by Adam and colleagues in 2004, in which 131 patients with 4 or more CRLM received neoadjuvant chemotherapy before hepatic resection. The 5-year DSS was 37% and 30% for those with responsive and stable disease, respectively. However, patients who progressed had a significantly worse DSS of 8%. This study concluded that patients who progress on neoadjuvant chemotherapy should not be offered resection. It is important that this study was performed on patients with extensive (>4 tumors) liver disease, many with extrahepatic metastases and many after second-line or third-line chemotherapy. Therefore, the findings of this study may not apply to patients with limited, liver-only resectable disease on first-line therapy. A recent study in a more modern cohort from MSKCC[83] has questioned these results. Neoadjuvant therapy led to a complete response in 6 patients and a partial response in 41 patients, while disease remained stable in 52 and progressed in 18. Five-year survival was 52%, and regardless of which response category the patients fell into, there was no significant difference in OS. Furthermore, there were no survival differences among the 3 response groups even when controlling for margins, stage, and CEA. Interestingly in this study, patients whose tumor progressed but who received HAI after resection demonstrated a trend toward better survival. Other more recent studies have also not shown differences in survival based on response or progression. A recent study by Neumann and colleagues[84] showed that among 160 patients undergoing complete resection of CRLM there was no difference in outcome based on response or progression with neoadjuvant chemotherapy. It must be stressed that these studies include patients progressing on chemotherapy only if selected for surgery and, so this small subset of patients is a highly selected group. Therefore, neoadjuvant therapy does not necessarily select patients for operative management and, even if patients progress on therapy and remain resectable, they still have the potential for long-term survival.

When neoadjuvant chemotherapy is being used to select patients for surgery, one must also consider the rate at which patients will progress while on modern chemotherapy. In the EORTC trial and other phase II trials,[85] the rate of progression is generally around 5%. Furthermore, in the EORTC trial 7% of patients progressed on preoperative chemotherapy, and some of these patients still underwent resection. Therefore, many patients would be receiving chemotherapy to theoretically select out a very small group of patients. One other argument to give chemotherapy preoperatively is that there can be failure to be able to deliver chemotherapy postoperatively because of complications of the surgery. Review of multiple prospective trials actually shows that the rate of adjuvant therapy delivered is fairly high and that the inability to deliver adjuvant chemotherapy is 5% to 23%. For example, the numbers of patients not receiving chemotherapy was 8 of 138 (5%) in the Mitry trial, 15 of 321 (5%) in the Ychou trial, and 36 of 151 (23%) in the EORTC perioperative chemotherapy arm[86–88] (of note, 8 of these were due to post-operative complications and 6 were due to toxic effects of pre-operative chemotherapy).[37,80,81]

Recent work has demonstrated that pathologic response has a prognostic role, and in a multi-institutional study of 171 patients undergoing resection of CRLM after preoperative chemotherapy, both pathologic response and tumor thickness at the tumor–normal liver interface were validated as predictors of DFS.[89] Preoperative chemotherapy and associated pathologic response were also evaluated in a series of 366 patients, and an overall pathologic response of greater than 75% and fibrosis greater than 40% were independently correlated to DSS.[90] Some liver metastases disappear on serial imaging during chemotherapy, and the relationship between this "radiologic complete response" and a pathologic response can be uncertain. In an initial study by Benoist and colleagues,[91] only 17% of radiologic complete responses (CRs) were true CR (pathologic CR or durable radiologic CR). However, a study by Auer and colleagues[16] looking at 435 CRLM patients showed that disappearing liver metastases (DLMs) after chemotherapy represented a true complete response in 66% of the cases and that HAIP use, inability to see these DLMs on MRI, and a normalized CEA were all independently associated with a true complete response. Although a radiologic CR is not completely reliable and generally all sites of disease should be resected among patients selected for surgery, use of MRI and disappearance while on HAI chemotherapy can help determine the likelihood of a true CR.

Neoadjuvant chemotherapy also has the potential to increase the morbidity of hepatic resection. Vauthey and colleagues[92] demonstrated that the rates of sinusoidal dilatation and steatohepatitis were 19% for oxaliplatin and 20% for irinotecan, and the resultant hepatic injury was associated with an increased mortality (6.5% vs 1.6%). In addition, the patients in the EORTC trial who received preoperative FOLFOX had a modestly increased morbidity.[88] In a recent publication from MSKCC, 384 patients undergoing hepatectomy for CRLM from 2003 to 2007 were evaluated for the association between preoperative chemotherapy and perioperative morbidity. Major postoperative complications were independently associated with 3 or more segment resections and perioperative blood transfusion, but not with preoperative chemotherapy or specific pathologic damage to hepatic parenchyma. These data contrast significantly with those from other studies such as that by Vauthey and colleagues[92] and the EORTC trial. These outcomes may be more reflective of patient selection and avoidance of major hepatic resections when there is evidence of significant hepatic damage.

Given these data, for patients with resectable disease the surgeon and medical oncologist should consider proceeding with a safe and potentially curative resection. Additional chemotherapy may improve PFS but has not been proved to increase OS. Additional chemotherapy can be given postoperatively, and when given preoperatively does not truly identify active agents and is not an efficient method of selecting patients for resection. Furthermore, preoperative chemotherapy may increase the risk of resection. Although there are many proponents of neoadjuvant chemotherapy, the authors believe that it is difficult to recommend its routine use in patients with limited and resectable CRLM.

CONVERSION CHEMOTHERAPY: DOWNSTAGING TO COMPLETE RESECTION

Given the outcomes after complete resection, it is unfortunate that only 10% to 20% of patients with CRLM are considered suitable candidates for hepatic metastasectomy.[93] With the major improvements in response rates with modern chemotherapy, many patients can be downstaged from initially unresectable disease to be considered potentially resectable. One of the most significant initial reports on this topic came from Paul Brousse Hospital, and reported on 1104 initially unresectable patients from 1988 to 1999. The study demonstrated that 12.5% of patients were downstaged and able to be taken to resection.[94] Survival among the downstaged patients was an encouraging 33% and 23% at 5 and 10 years. Although this was somewhat worse than those patients who were initially resectable (48% and 30%), the outcomes were encouraging and showed that long-term survival was possible.[94] These data strongly suggested that selected patients with unresectable disease and with response to chemotherapy can realize a survival benefit. Other studies have demonstrated that unresectable metastases can become resectable using systemic chemotherapy. Both retrospective reviews and prospective trials on systemic therapy have documented conversion to complete resection, with rates ranging from 10% to 60%.[95–97] Most of these studies also document that resected patients have outcomes similar to those of patients who were initially resectable, with a significant chance for long-term survival and even the potential for cure. One of the major issues is that the definition of resectability is complex, involves biological and technical issues, and is extremely variable between institutions. This aspect probably accounts for the large variation in conversion to resection.

HAI chemotherapy has also been a promising treatment for conversion of patients to complete resection. A phase I trial using HAI with FUDR and systemic irinotecan and oxaliplatin in 49 patients with unresectable CRLM was reviewed to determine the resectability rate in 49 patients.[98] All 49 patients were re-reviewed to demonstrate technically unresectable disease with extensive parenchymal and vascular involvement. Patients generally had very advanced malignancy, with 90% having a CRS of 3 or more and 53% having been previously treated. Overall, 92% had a complete or partial response and 47% were converted to complete resection (**Fig. 3**).[98] Given that this initial report was a retrospective review, the authors performed a prospective phase II study in 49 patients with unresectable CRLM to document these outcomes in the context of a clear definition of resectability. Treatment consisted of HAI with FUDR, best systemic chemotherapy, and bevacizumab. Patients in this trial had very advanced CRLM with a median of 14 tumors. Furthermore, 65% of patients had been previously treated. A 76% response rate was noted, and 23 (47%) converted to resection. Conversion to resection was the only factor associated with longer OS and PFS on multivariate analysis. In a landmark analysis, resected patients had a 3-year survival of 80% compared with 26% for those who could not undergo resection. Most importantly, 10 patients (20%) were free of disease at a median follow-up of 39 months. Of note, in this trial a high degree of biliary complications were noted in the first 24 patients, and bevacizumab was discontinued for the last 25 patients in the study following improvement in the biliary toxicity.

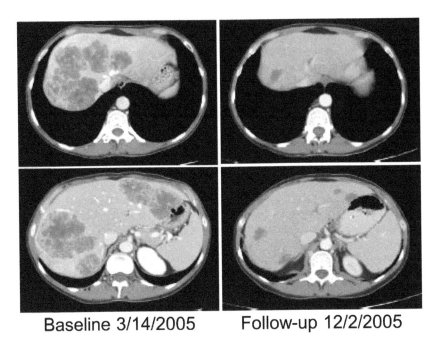

Baseline 3/14/2005   Follow-up 12/2/2005

Fig. 3. Conversion to resectability with hepatic artery infusion (HAI) and systemic chemotherapy. Computed tomography scans from a representative patient with extensive disease with vascular involvement are shown both pre- and post-HAI plus chemotherapy. This patient was converted to a resectable state after HAI and systemic chemotherapy. Of note, the carcinoembryonic antigen level went from 156 to 2.9 ng/mL, and the patient had no evidence of recurrence 2 years status post resection. (*Adapted from* Kemeny NE, Melendez FD, Capanu M, et al. Conversion to resectability using hepatic artery infusion plus systemic chemotherapy for the treatment of unresectable liver metastases from colorectal carcinoma. J Clin Oncol 2009;27(21):3465–71; with permission.)

In summary, conversion to complete resection is a reasonable goal for patients with unresectable CRLM. Both systemic and combined HAI therapy show promising results. Most studies do a poor job of defining resectability, making the data difficult to interpret. Nonetheless, in an otherwise healthy patient, serious consideration should be given to resection in patients with advanced disease and good response to chemotherapy.

RE-RESECTION FOR RECURRENCE OF COLORECTAL LIVER METASTASES

Before 1994, the role of repeat resection for recurrent CRLM was not an established treatment modality. Approximately 8 reports had been published describing re-resection; however, none of these were able to make a strong case for its role.[99–106] Fong and colleagues[107] set out to determine if repeat liver resections for CRLM justified the potential morbidity inherent in these cases. Over the course of 6 years, 499 patients underwent liver resection for CRLM at MSKCC, and 44 of these patients were re-explored for presumed liver recurrence, 25 of whom were able to be resected. No in-hospital or 30-day mortality was observed and morbidity occurred in 28%, comparing favorably with previous reports (range 15%[100]–50%[104]). The median DFS was 9 months after the second resection, compared with 12 months for the first liver resection. Eleven patients were 2-year survivors, but no 5-year survivors were noted at the time of the study. This initial report documented that re-resection was feasible but that long-term oncologic efficacy remained unproven. Pinson and colleagues[108] subsequently reported on a series of 10 of 95 patients from a similar time period who underwent re-resection for recurrent hepatic disease. There was no operative mortality, but morbidity was 60%; at a mean follow-up of 33 months no deaths had occurred, and DFS was 60% and 45% at 1 and 3 years, respectively. Sixty percent of the patients developed re-recurrence after repeat hepatectomy at a median of 9 months, and 20% underwent a third hepatectomy. In 2002, experience at MSKCC was combined with the University of Frankfurt, and a total of 126 patients were evaluated who underwent repeat hepatectomy for recurrent CRLM from 1985 to 2001.[109] Median follow-up after the second liver operation was 59 months. Two patients died within 30 days of operation, and the morbidity rate was 28%. The median OS was 37 months, and significantly better survival was noted for patients with solitary and/or small tumors. These data demonstrate that repeat liver resections are safe, and in well-selected patients can be associated with prolonged survival.

SUMMARY

The surgical management of CRLM is complex. The interplay between appropriate diagnosis and workup, surgical technique, perioperative management, perioperative chemotherapy, and the defining role of tumor biology make this a fascinating field of study and practice. The argument for hepatic resection is supported by the fact that patients are cured by surgery at a rate similar to that for some primary nonmetastatic malignancies. The goal of surgery should be to obtain an R0 resection and, although nonanatomic wedge resections are sometimes sufficient, wider segmental or lobar resections may provide a better chance of surgical success. Overall the rate of operative resectability is high, and a small minority of patients undergoes nontherapeutic laparotomy. Predictors of survival include size and number of tumors, short disease-free interval, node-positive primary tumor, positive margins, and the presence of EHD. These factors do not always exclude patients from resection given the possibility of long-term survival, even in the presence of poor prognostic factors. Molecular and immunologic markers will play a role in even better selection of patients led by biology.

Overall mortality after hepatic resection for CRLM at major United States centers is less than 1%, likely resulting from improved operative technique and patient selection. Recognition and appropriate management of postoperative morbidity still plays a significant role in the care of these patients, but with the use of parenchymal-sparing techniques and low CVP anesthesia in addition to specialized care in tertiary centers, these rates are acceptable. Systemic chemotherapy has improved for patients with unresectable CRLM, but randomized trials to date have not shown a significant improvement in outcomes with modern regimens given in the perioperative setting. Response to neoadjuvant therapy is not a defining measure, as even patients with progression who remain resectable can enjoy long-term survival after resection. Conversion to complete resection can be obtained in patients with unresectable CRLM using a combination of systemic and HAI therapy. Finally, re-resection of recurrent disease is safe and can be beneficial in carefully selected patients.

REFERENCES

1. Valastyan S, Weinberg RA. Tumor metastasis: molecular insights and evolving paradigms. Cell 2011;147(2):275–92.

2. Jemal A, Center MM, DeSantis C, et al. Global patterns of cancer incidence and mortality rates and trends. Cancer Epidemiol Biomarkers Prev 2010;19(8):1893–907.

3. Siegel R, Ma J, Zou Z, et al. Cancer statistics, 2014. CA Cancer J Clin 2014; 64(1):9–29.

4. Tzeng CW, Aloia TA. Colorectal liver metastases. J Gastrointest Surg 2013; 17(1):195–201 [quiz: 201–2].

5. Fong Y, Fortner J, Sun RL, et al. Clinical score for predicting recurrence after hepatic resection for metastatic colorectal cancer: analysis of 1001 consecutive cases. Ann Surg 1999;230(3):309–18 [discussion: 318–21].

6. Stangl R, Altendorf-Hofmann A, Charnley RM, et al. Factors influencing the natural history of colorectal liver metastases. Lancet 1994;343(8910):1405–10.

7. Tomlinson JS, Jarnagin WR, DeMatteo RP, et al. Actual 10-year survival after resection of colorectal liver metastases defines cure. J Clin Oncol 2007; 25(29):4575–80.

8. Foster JH, Berman M. Solid liver tumors. Philadelphia: W.B. Saunders Company; 1977.

9. Scheele J, Stangl R, Altendorf-Hofmann A. Hepatic metastases from colorectal carcinoma: impact of surgical resection on the natural history. Br J Surg 1990; 77(11):1241–6.

10. Choti MA, Sitzmann JV, Tiburi MF, et al. Trends in long-term survival following liver resection for hepatic colorectal metastases. Ann Surg 2002;235(6):759–66.

11. Brouquet A, Abdalla EK, Kopetz S, et al. High survival rate after two-stage resection of advanced colorectal liver metastases: response-based selection and complete resection define outcome. J Clin Oncol 2011;29(8):1083–90.

12. Gallagher DJ, Kemeny N. Metastatic colorectal cancer: from improved survival to potential cure. Oncology 2010;78(3–4):237–48.

13. Silen W. Hepatic resection for metastases from colorectal carcinoma is of dubious value. Arch Surg 1989;124(9):1021–2.

14. Benson AB 3rd, Bekaii-Saab T, Chan E, et al. Metastatic colon cancer, version 3.2013: featured updates to the NCCN Guidelines. J Natl Compr Canc Netw 2013;11(2):141–52 [quiz: 152].

15. Poultsides GA, Servais EL, Saltz LB, et al. Outcome of primary tumor in patients with synchronous stage IV colorectal cancer receiving combination chemotherapy without surgery as initial treatment. J Clin Oncol 2009;27(20):3379–84.

16. Auer RC, White RR, Kemeny NE, et al. Predictors of a true complete response among disappearing liver metastases from colorectal cancer after chemotherapy. Cancer 2010;116(6):1502–9.

17. Fong Y, Saldinger PF, Akhurst T, et al. Utility of ^{18}F-FDG positron emission tomography scanning on selection of patients for resection of hepatic colorectal metastases. Am J Surg 1999;178(4):282–7.

18. Lejeune C, Bismuth MJ, Conroy T, et al. Use of a decision analysis model to assess the cost-effectiveness of ^{18}F-FDG PET in the management of metachronous liver metastases of colorectal cancer. J Nucl Med 2005;46(12):2020–8.

19. Moulton CA, Gu CS, Law CH, et al. Effect of PET before liver resection on surgical management for colorectal adenocarcinoma metastases: a randomized clinical trial. JAMA 2014;311(18):1863–9.

20. Benson AB 3rd, Bekaii-Saab T, Chan E, et al. Localized colon cancer, version 3.2013: featured updates to the NCCN Guidelines. J Natl Compr Canc Netw 2013;11(5):519–28.

21. Frankel TL, D'Angelica MI. Hepatic resection for colorectal metastases. J Surg Oncol 2014;109(1):2–7.

22. Ekberg H, Tranberg KG, Andersson R, et al. Determinants of survival in liver resection for colorectal secondaries. Br J Surg 1986;73(9):727–31.
23. D'Angelica M. Are patients with multiple hepatic metastases from colorectal cancer candidates for surgery? Nature clinical practice. Oncology 2007;4(12):682–3.
24. Cady B, Stone MD, McDermott WV Jr, et al. Technical and biological factors in disease-free survival after hepatic resection for colorectal cancer metastases. Arch Surg 1992;127(5):561–8 [discussion: 568–9].
25. Weber SM, Jarnagin WR, DeMatteo RP, et al. Survival after resection of multiple hepatic colorectal metastases. Ann Surg Oncol 2000;7(9):643–50.
26. Pawlik TM, Abdalla EK, Ellis LM, et al. Debunking dogma: surgery for four or more colorectal liver metastases is justified. J Gastrointest Surg 2006;10(2):240–8.
27. Kornprat P, Jarnagin WR, Gonen M, et al. Outcome after hepatectomy for multiple (four or more) colorectal metastases in the era of effective chemotherapy. Ann Surg Oncol 2007;14(3):1151–60.
28. Malik HZ, Hamady ZZ, Adair R, et al. Prognostic influence of multiple hepatic metastases from colorectal cancer. Eur J Surg Oncol 2007;33(4):468–73.
29. Cady B, Jenkins RL, Steele GD Jr, et al. Surgical margin in hepatic resection for colorectal metastasis: a critical and improvable determinant of outcome. Ann Surg 1998;227(4):566–71.
30. Pawlik TM, Scoggins CR, Zorzi D, et al. Effect of surgical margin status on survival and site of recurrence after hepatic resection for colorectal metastases. Ann Surg 2005;241(5):715–22 [discussion: 722–4].
31. Are C, Gonen M, Zazzali K, et al. The impact of margins on outcome after hepatic resection for colorectal metastasis. Ann Surg 2007;246(2):295–300.
32. DeMatteo RP, Palese C, Jarnagin WR, et al. Anatomic segmental hepatic resection is superior to wedge resection as an oncologic operation for colorectal liver metastases. J Gastrointest Surg 2000;4(2):178–84.
33. Blumgart LH, Fong Y. Surgical options in the treatment of hepatic metastasis from colorectal cancer. Curr Probl Surg 1995;32(5):333–421.
34. Elias D, Liberale G, Vernerey D, et al. Hepatic and extrahepatic colorectal metastases: when resectable, their localization does not matter, but their total number has a prognostic effect. Ann Surg Oncol 2005;12(11):900–9.
35. Carpizo DR, D'Angelica M. Liver resection for metastatic colorectal cancer in the presence of extrahepatic disease. Ann Surg Oncol 2009;16(9):2411–21.
36. Jarnagin WR, Fong Y, Ky A, et al. Liver resection for metastatic colorectal cancer: assessing the risk of occult irresectable disease. J Am Coll Surg 1999;188(1):33–42.
37. Grobmyer SR, Fong Y, D'Angelica M, et al. Diagnostic laparoscopy prior to planned hepatic resection for colorectal metastases. Arch Surg 2004;139(12):1326–30.
38. Bickenbach KA, Dematteo RP, Fong Y, et al. Risk of occult irresectable disease at liver resection for hepatic colorectal cancer metastases: a contemporary analysis. Ann Surg Oncol 2013;20(6):2029–34.
39. Martin R, Paty P, Fong Y, et al. Simultaneous liver and colorectal resections are safe for synchronous colorectal liver metastasis. J Am Coll Surg 2003;197(2):233–41 [discussion: 241–2].
40. Reddy SK, Pawlik TM, Zorzi D, et al. Simultaneous resections of colorectal cancer and synchronous liver metastases: a multi-institutional analysis. Ann Surg Oncol 2007;14(12):3481–91.

41. Hillingso JG, Wille-Jorgensen P. Staged or simultaneous resection of synchronous liver metastases from colorectal cancer–a systematic review. Colorectal Dis 2009;11(1):3–10.
42. Rougier P, Milan C, Lazorthes F, et al. Prospective study of prognostic factors in patients with unresected hepatic metastases from colorectal cancer. Fondation Francaise de Cancerologie Digestive. Br J Surg 1995;82(10):1397–400.
43. Manfredi S, Lepage C, Hatem C, et al. Epidemiology and management of liver metastases from colorectal cancer. Ann Surg 2006;244(2):254–9.
44. Kopetz S, Chang GJ, Overman MJ, et al. Improved survival in metastatic colorectal cancer is associated with adoption of hepatic resection and improved chemotherapy. J Clin Oncol 2009;27(22):3677–83.
45. House MG, Ito H, Gonen M, et al. Survival after hepatic resection for metastatic colorectal cancer: trends in outcomes for 1,600 patients during two decades at a single institution. J Am Coll Surg 2010;210(5):744–52, 752–5.
46. Zakaria S, Donohue JH, Que FG, et al. Hepatic resection for colorectal metastases: value for risk scoring systems? Ann Surg 2007;246(2):183–91.
47. Kattan MW, Gonen M, Jarnagin WR, et al. A nomogram for predicting disease-specific survival after hepatic resection for metastatic colorectal cancer. Ann Surg 2008;247(2):282–7.
48. Takakura Y, Okajima M, Kanemitsu Y, et al. External validation of two nomograms for predicting patient survival after hepatic resection for metastatic colorectal cancer. World J Surg 2011;35(10):2275–82.
49. Kattan MW, Marasco J. What is a real nomogram? Semin Oncol 2010;37(1):23–6.
50. Ito H, Mo Q, Qin LX, et al. Gene expression profiles accurately predict outcome following liver resection in patients with metastatic colorectal cancer. PLoS One 2013;8(12):e81680.
51. Wong VK, Malik HZ, Hamady ZZ, et al. C-reactive protein as a predictor of prognosis following curative resection for colorectal liver metastases. Br J Cancer 2007;96(2):222–5.
52. Kishi Y, Kopetz S, Chun YS, et al. Blood neutrophil-to-lymphocyte ratio predicts survival in patients with colorectal liver metastases treated with systemic chemotherapy. Ann Surg Oncol 2009;16(3):614–22.
53. Katz SC, Pillarisetty V, Bamboat ZM, et al. T cell infiltrate predicts long-term survival following resection of colorectal cancer liver metastases. Ann Surg Oncol 2009;16(9):2524–30.
54. Yopp AC, Shia J, Butte JM, et al. CXCR4 expression predicts patient outcome and recurrence patterns after hepatic resection for colorectal liver metastases. Ann Surg Oncol 2012;19(Suppl 3):S339–46.
55. Tan MC, Butte JM, Gonen M, et al. Prognostic significance of early recurrence: a conditional survival analysis in patients with resected colorectal liver metastasis. HPB (Oxford) 2013;15(10):803–13.
56. Foster JH. Survival after liver resection for cancer. Cancer 1970;26(3):493–502.
57. Aloia TA, Fahy BN, Fischer CP, et al. Predicting poor outcome following hepatectomy: analysis of 2313 hepatectomies in the NSQIP database. HPB (Oxford) 2009;11(6):510–5.
58. Andres A, Toso C, Moldovan B, et al. Complications of elective liver resections in a center with low mortality: a simple score to predict morbidity. Arch Surg 2011; 146(11):1246–52.
59. Ito H, Are C, Gonen M, et al. Effect of postoperative morbidity on long-term survival after hepatic resection for metastatic colorectal cancer. Ann Surg 2008; 247(6):994–1002.

60. Matsuda A, Matsumoto S, Seya T, et al. Does postoperative complication have a negative impact on long-term outcomes following hepatic resection for colorectal liver metastasis?: a meta-analysis. Ann Surg Oncol 2013;20(8):2485–92.
61. Gold JS, Are C, Kornprat P, et al. Increased use of parenchymal-sparing surgery for bilateral liver metastases from colorectal cancer is associated with improved mortality without change in oncologic outcome: trends in treatment over time in 440 patients. Ann Surg 2008;247(1):109–17.
62. Scheele J, Stang R, Altendorf-Hofmann A, et al. Resection of colorectal liver metastases. World J Surg 1995;19(1):59–71.
63. Man K, Fan ST, Ng IO, et al. Prospective evaluation of Pringle maneuver in hepatectomy for liver tumors by a randomized study. Ann Surg 1997;226(6):704–11 [discussion: 711–3].
64. Belghiti J, Noun R, Zante E, et al. Portal triad clamping or hepatic vascular exclusion for major liver resection. A controlled study. Ann Surg 1996;224(2):155–61.
65. Stephenson KR, Steinberg SM, Hughes KS, et al. Perioperative blood transfusions are associated with decreased time to recurrence and decreased survival after resection of colorectal liver metastases. Ann Surg 1988;208(6):679–87.
66. Rosen CB, Nagorney DM, Taswell HF, et al. Perioperative blood transfusion and determinants of survival after liver resection for metastatic colorectal carcinoma. Ann Surg 1992;216(4):493–504 [discussion: 504–5].
67. Kooby DA, Stockman J, Ben-Porat L, et al. Influence of transfusions on perioperative and long-term outcome in patients following hepatic resection for colorectal metastases. Ann Surg 2003;237(6):860–9 [discussion: 869–70].
68. Melendez JA, Arslan V, Fischer ME, et al. Perioperative outcomes of major hepatic resections under low central venous pressure anesthesia: blood loss, blood transfusion, and the risk of postoperative renal dysfunction. J Am Coll Surg 1998;187(6):620–5.
69. Jarnagin WR, Gonen M, Maithel SK, et al. A prospective randomized trial of acute normovolemic hemodilution compared to standard intraoperative management in patients undergoing major hepatic resection. Ann Surg 2008; 248(3):360–9.
70. Adson MA, van Heerden JA, Adson MH, et al. Resection of hepatic metastases from colorectal cancer. Arch Surg 1984;119(6):647–51.
71. McCormack PM, Burt ME, Bains MS, et al. Lung resection for colorectal metastases. 10-year results. Arch Surg 1992;127(12):1403–6.
72. Miller G, Biernacki P, Kemeny NE, et al. Outcomes after resection of synchronous or metachronous hepatic and pulmonary colorectal metastases. J Am Coll Surg 2007;205(2):231–8.
73. Maithel SK, Ginsberg MS, D'Amico F, et al. Natural history of patients with subcentimeter pulmonary nodules undergoing hepatic resection for metastatic colorectal cancer. J Am Coll Surg 2010;210(1):31–8.
74. Nordlinger B, Sorbye H, Glimelius B, et al. Perioperative FOLFOX4 chemotherapy and surgery versus surgery alone for resectable liver metastases from colorectal cancer (EORTC 40983): long-term results of a randomised, controlled, phase 3 trial. Lancet Oncol 2013;14(12):1208–15.
75. Primrose J, Falk S, Finch-Jones M, et al. Systemic chemotherapy with or without cetuximab in patients with resectable colorectal liver metastasis: the New EPOC randomised controlled trial. Lancet Oncol 2014;15(6):601–11.
76. Ensminger WD, Rosowsky A, Raso V, et al. A clinical-pharmacological evaluation of hepatic arterial infusions of 5-fluoro-2'-deoxyuridine and 5-fluorouracil. Cancer Res 1978;38(11 Pt 1):3784–92.

77. Kemeny N, Jarnagin W, Gonen M, et al. Phase I/II study of hepatic arterial therapy with floxuridine and dexamethasone in combination with intravenous irinotecan as adjuvant treatment after resection of hepatic metastases from colorectal cancer. J Clin Oncol 2003;21(17):3303–9.
78. Kemeny NE, Gonen M. Hepatic arterial infusion after liver resection. N Engl J Med 2005;352(7):734–5.
79. Sigurdson ER, Ridge JA, Kemeny N, et al. Tumor and liver drug uptake following hepatic artery and portal vein infusion. J Clin Oncol 1987;5(11):1836–40.
80. House MG, Kemeny NE, Gonen M, et al. Comparison of adjuvant systemic chemotherapy with or without hepatic arterial infusional chemotherapy after hepatic resection for metastatic colorectal cancer. Ann Surg 2011;254(6):851–6.
81. Kemeny NE, Jarnagin WR, Capanu M, et al. Randomized phase II trial of adjuvant hepatic arterial infusion and systemic chemotherapy with or without bevacizumab in patients with resected hepatic metastases from colorectal cancer. J Clin Oncol 2011;29(7):884–9.
82. Ito K, Ito H, Kemeny NE, et al. Biliary sclerosis after hepatic arterial infusion pump chemotherapy for patients with colorectal cancer liver metastasis: incidence, clinical features, and risk factors. Ann Surg Oncol 2012;19(5):1609–17.
83. Gallagher DJ, Zheng J, Capanu M, et al. Response to neoadjuvant chemotherapy does not predict survival for patients with synchronous colorectal hepatic metastases. Ann Surg Oncol 2009;16(7):1844–51.
84. Neumann UP, Thelan A, Rocken C, et al. Nonresponse to preoperative chemotherapy does not preclude long-term survival after liver resection in patients with colorectal liver metastases. Surgery 2009;146(1):52–9.
85. Gruenberger B, Tamandl D, Schueller J, et al. Bevacizumab, capecitabine, and oxaliplatin as neoadjuvant therapy for patients with potentially curable metastatic colorectal cancer. J Clin Oncol 2008;26(11):1830–5.
86. Mitry E, Fields AL, Bleiberg H, et al. Adjuvant chemotherapy after potentially curative resection of metastases from colorectal cancer: a pooled analysis of two randomized trials. J Clin Oncol 2008;26(30):4906–11.
87. Ychou M, Hohenberger W, Thezenas S, et al. A randomized phase III study comparing adjuvant 5-fluorouracil/folinic acid with FOLFIRI in patients following complete resection of liver metastases from colorectal cancer. Ann Oncol 2009; 20(12):1964–70.
88. Nordlinger B, Sorbye H, Glimelius B, et al. Perioperative chemotherapy with FOLFOX4 and surgery versus surgery alone for resectable liver metastases from colorectal cancer (EORTC Intergroup trial 40983): a randomised controlled trial. Lancet 2008;371(9617):1007–16.
89. Brouquet A, Zimmitti G, Kopetz S, et al. Multicenter validation study of pathologic response and tumor thickness at the tumor-normal liver interface as independent predictors of disease-free survival after preoperative chemotherapy and surgery for colorectal liver metastases. Cancer 2013;119(15):2778–88.
90. Poultsides GA, Bao F, Servais EL, et al. Pathologic response to preoperative chemotherapy in colorectal liver metastases: fibrosis, not necrosis, predicts outcome. Ann Surg Oncol 2012;19(9):2797–804.
91. Benoist S, Brouquet A, Penna C, et al. Complete response of colorectal liver metastases after chemotherapy: does it mean cure? J Clin Oncol 2006;24(24):3939–45.
92. Vauthey JN, Pawlik TM, Ribero D, et al. Chemotherapy regimen predicts steatohepatitis and an increase in 90-day mortality after surgery for hepatic colorectal metastases. J Clin Oncol 2006;24(13):2065–72.

93. Jarnagin WR, Conlon K, Bodniewicz J, et al. A clinical scoring system predicts the yield of diagnostic laparoscopy in patients with potentially resectable hepatic colorectal metastases. Cancer 2001;91(6):1121–8.

94. Adam R, Delvart V, Pascal G, et al. Rescue surgery for unresectable colorectal liver metastases downstaged by chemotherapy: a model to predict long-term survival. Ann Surg 2004;240(4):644–57 [discussion: 657–8].

95. Adam R, Avisar E, Ariche A, et al. Five-year survival following hepatic resection after neoadjuvant therapy for nonresectable colorectal. Ann Surg Oncol 2001; 8(4):347–53.

96. Bismuth H, Adam R, Levi F, et al. Resection of nonresectable liver metastases from colorectal cancer after neoadjuvant chemotherapy. Ann Surg 1996; 224(4):509–20 [discussion: 520–2].

97. Jones RP, Hamann S, Malik HZ, et al. Defined criteria for resectability improves rates of secondary resection after systemic therapy for liver limited metastatic colorectal cancer. Eur J Cancer 2014;50(9):1590–601.

98. Kemeny NE, Melendez FD, Capanu M, et al. Conversion to resectability using hepatic artery infusion plus systemic chemotherapy for the treatment of unresectable liver metastases from colorectal carcinoma. J Clin Oncol 2009; 27(21):3465–71.

99. Vaillant JC, Balladur P, Nordlinger B, et al. Repeat liver resection for recurrent colorectal metastases. Br J Surg 1993;80(3):340–4.

100. Lange JF, Leese T, Castaing D, et al. Repeat hepatectomy for recurrent malignant tumors of the liver. Surg Gynecol Obstet 1989;169(2):119–26.

101. Hohenberger P, Schlag P, Schwarz V, et al. Tumor recurrence and options for further treatment after resection of liver metastases in patients with colorectal cancer. J Surg Oncol 1990;44(4):245–51.

102. Griffith KD, Sugarbaker PH, Chang AE. Repeat hepatic resections for colorectal metastases. Surgery 1990;107(1):101–4.

103. Butler J, Attiyeh FF, Daly JM. Hepatic resection for metastases of the colon and rectum. Surg Gynecol Obstet 1986;162(2):109–13.

104. Bozzetti F, Bignami P, Montalto F, et al. Repeated hepatic resection for recurrent metastases from colorectal cancer. Br J Surg 1992;79(2):146–8.

105. Fortner JG. Recurrence of colorectal cancer after hepatic resection. Am J Surg 1988;155(3):378–82.

106. Nordlinger B, Quilichini MA, Parc R, et al. Hepatic resection for colorectal liver metastases. Influence on survival of preoperative factors and surgery for recurrences in 80 patients. Ann Surg 1987;205(3):256–63.

107. Fong Y, Blumgart LH, Cohen A, et al. Repeat hepatic resections for metastatic colorectal cancer. Ann Surg 1994;220(5):657–62.

108. Pinson CW, Wright JK, Chapman WC, et al. Repeat hepatic surgery for colorectal cancer metastasis to the liver. Ann Surg 1996;223(6):765–73 [discussion: 773–6].

109. Petrowsky H, Gonen M, Jarnagin W, et al. Second liver resections are safe and effective treatment for recurrent hepatic metastases from colorectal cancer: a bi-institutional analysis. Ann Surg 2002;235(6):863–71.

110. Hughes KS, Simon R, Songhorabodi S, et al. Resection of the liver for colorectal carcinoma metastases: a multi-institutional study of patterns of recurrence. Surgery 1986;100(2):278–84.

111. Scheele J, Stangl R, Altendorf-Hofmann A, et al. Indicators of prognosis after hepatic resection for colorectal secondaries. Surgery 1991;110(1):13–29.

112. Gayowski TJ, Iwatsuki S, Madariaga JR, et al. Experience in hepatic resection for metastatic colorectal cancer: analysis of clinical and pathologic risk factors. Surgery 1994;116(4):703–10.
113. Nordlinger B, Guiguet M, Vaillant JC, et al. Surgical resection of colorectal carcinoma metastases to the liver. A prognostic scoring system to improve case selection, based on 1568 patients. Association Française de Chirurgie. Cancer 1996;77(7):1254–62.
114. Jamison RL, Donohue JH, Nagorney DM, et al. Hepatic resection for metastatic colorectal cancer results in cure for some patients. Arch Surg 1997;132(5): 505–10.
115. Abdulla EK, Vauthey JN, Ellis LM, et al. Recurrence and outcomes following hepatic resection, radiofrequency ablation, and combined resection/ablation for colorectal liver metastases. Ann Surg 2004;239(6):818–25.

Is More Not Better?
Combination Therapies in Colorectal Cancer Treatment

Emily K. Bergsland, MD

KEYWORDS

- Combination chemotherapy • Adjuvant therapy • Targeted therapy
- First-line therapy • Metastatic colorectal cancer • Systemic therapy
- Optimal sequence

KEY POINTS

- The availability of new chemotherapeutic agents (oxaliplatin, irinotecan, capecitabine) as well as vascular endothelial growth factor and epidermal growth factor receptor inhibitors has translated into improved outcomes in colorectal cancer (CRC).
- With respect to combination therapy for CRC, more is often better, but at the expense of increased toxicity and cost. It also has the potential to lead to worse outcomes, underscoring the importance of randomized clinical trials and appropriate patient selection.
- The addition of oxaliplatin improves outcomes in stage III colon cancer, but the data do not support its use in stage II colon cancer, patients older than 70 years, or as a radiosensitizer in rectal cancer. Furthermore, targeted agents have no role in adjuvant therapy for colon cancer.
- Choice of therapy for metastatic disease is governed by several factors, including previous therapy, comorbidities, goals of therapy, tumor mutational status, and personal preference.
- The small incremental benefits observed with individual lines of therapy will hopefully be enhanced by better patient selection (ie, avoiding unnecessary toxicity in patients who are unlikely to benefit and accepting toxicity in patients who stand to benefit the most from combination therapy).

INTRODUCTION

The treatment of colorectal cancer has evolved dramatically over the last decade, as shown by the availability of additional chemotherapeutic agents as well as agents targeting the vascular endothelial growth factor (VEGF)–signaling and epidermal

Department of Medicine, Division of Hematology and Oncology, UCSF Helen Diller Family Comprehensive Cancer Center, 1600 Divisadero Street, A727, San Francisco, CA 94115, USA
E-mail address: emilyb@medicine.ucsf.edu

Hematol Oncol Clin N Am 29 (2015) 85–116
http://dx.doi.org/10.1016/j.hoc.2014.09.002
0889-8588/15/$ – see front matter © 2015 Elsevier Inc. All rights reserved.

hemonc.theclinics.com

growth factor receptor (EGFR)-signaling pathways. The most striking impact has been in patients with metastatic disease, in whom access to these new therapeutic strategies has been associated with a more than doubling of overall survival (OS). Although more has often translated into better (eg, higher response rates [RRs] with combination chemotherapy), more has also typically come at a price, both literally and figuratively, leading one to question if more is always better, and if some patients stand to benefit more than others. This issue is perhaps best exemplified by the lack of incremental benefit of greater than 6 months of adjuvant chemotherapy for stage III colon cancer, the lack of benefit from targeted agents in the adjuvant setting, and the potential for harm when EGFR inhibitors are used in patients with RAS mutant tumors or when combining targeted agents for first-line treatment of metastatic disease. Furthermore, less may be acceptable in the setting of maintenance therapy for advanced disease, but giving something may be better than nothing. Additional information is needed to optimize patient selection and choice of therapy in treating colorectal cancer.

ADJUVANT COMBINATION THERAPY FOR RESECTABLE COLON CANCER
Stage III Colon Cancer

Given a significant risk of recurrence, the use of adjuvant fluoropyrimidine (FP)-based treatment is standard in stage III colon cancer.[1,2] This treatment was initially given for 12 months, and subsequent studies proved that more was not superior to less. The optimal duration of therapy is unknown, but the data suggest that adjuvant therapy should not be given for more than 6 months.[3] Most of the current phase 3 trials in adjuvant therapy are focused on the optimal duration of therapy (**Table 1**), many of which are encompassed by the IDEA (International Duration Evaluation of Adjuvant Chemotherapy) collaboration.[4] In terms of combination chemotherapy (**Table 2**), the addition of oxaliplatin (OX) (eg, FOLFOX [infusional/bolus 5-fluorouracil, leucovorin, OX], XELOX [capecitabine (CAPE)/OX], FLOX [OX, bolus 5-fluorouracil, leucovorin]) improves disease-free survival (DFS) in patients with stage III disease.[5–7] In addition, in the Multicenter International Study of Oxaliplatin, 5-Fluorouracil, Leucovorin in the Adjuvant Treatment of Colon Cancer (MOSAIC) study, treatment with FOLFOX

Table 1
Adjuvant therapy for colon cancer: selected ongoing phase III trials[a]

Study ID	Stage	Study Arms	Location
CALGB/SWOG 80702	III	FOLFOX (3 vs 6 mo) with or without celecoxib	United States
ICOG-CC01	IIIA/B	UFT/LV with or without polysaccharide-K	Japan
2007-000354-31	II/III	FOLFOX (3 vs 6 mo) with or without bevacizumab	Italy
CDR0000613042	II/III	12 vs 6 cycles OxMdG or XELOX	UK
CDR0000647466	III	3 vs 6 mo FOLFOX or XELOX	France
2009-11-008	II/III	3 vs 6 mo of oxaliplatin in patients receiving 6 mo adjuvant FOLFOX/CAPOX	Korea
CT/09.12	II/III	3 vs 6 mo FOLFOX/CAPOX	Greece
NeoCol	T3,4	Neoadjuvant chemo × 3 followed by surgery vs surgery + adjuvant chemo × 8	Denmark

Abbreviations: CAPOX/XELOX, capecitabine/oxaliplatin; FOLFOX/OxMdG, infusional/bolus 5-fluorouracil, leucovorin, oxaliplatin; LV, leucovorin; UFT, tegafur-uracil.
   [a] http://www.clinicaltrials.gov.

Table 2
Results of selected phase 3 adjuvant trials with combination chemotherapy in colon cancer

Study	Stage	Study Arms	N	Primary Endpoint	DFS (%)	OS (%)	Reference
Oxaliplatin-Based							
MOSAIC	II/III	FOLFOX4 LV5FU2	2246	DFS	73.3 67.4 at 5 y; HR = 0.80; 95% CI, 0.68–0.93; P = .003	78.5 76 at 6 y; HR = 0.84; 95% CI, 0.71 to 1.00; P = .046	Andre et al,[6] 2009
	II/III					No Change 68.7/72.9, HR = 0.80; 95% CI, 0.65 to 0.97; P = .023	Andre et al,[6] 2009
NSABP C07	II/III	FLOX FU/LV	2407	DFS	73.2 67.0 at 4 y; HR = 0.80; 95% CI, 0.69–0.93; P<.004	No change	Kuebler et al,[8] 2007
NO16968	III	XELOX FU/LV	1886	DFS	70.9 66.5 at 3 y; HR = 0.80; 95% CI, 0.69–0.93; P = .0045	No change (77.6/74.2 at 5 y)	Haller et al,[7] 2011
Irinotecan-Based							
FNCLCC Accord02/ FFCD9802	III	FOLFIRI LV5FU2	400	DFS	No change	No change	Ychou et al,[11] 2009
CALGB 89803	III	IFL FU/LV	1264	OS, DFS	No change	No change	Saltz et al,[12] 2007
PETACC-3	III	FOLFIRI LV5FU2	2094	DFS	No change at 5 y	No change at 5 y (73.6/71.3)	Van Cutsem et al,[13] 2009

Abbreviations: CI, confidence interval; DFS, disease-free survival; FLOX, oxaliplatin, bolus 5-fluorouracil, leucovorin; FOLFIRI, infusional/bolus fluorouracil, leucovorin, irinotecan; FOLFOX, infusional/bolus 5-fluorouracil, leucovorin, oxaliplatin; FU, 5-fluorouracil; HR, hazard ratio; IFL, bolus irinotecan, 5-flurouracil, leucovorin; LV, leucovorin; LV5FU2, infusional/bolus 5-fluorouracil, leucovorin; OS, overall survival; XELOX, capecitabine/oxaliplatin.

improved OS at 6 years in stage III patients (72.9% vs 68.7%; hazard ratio [HR] = 0.8; 95% confidence interval [CI], 0.65–0.97; P = .023). The incremental benefit of OX-based therapy comes at a price (eg, hand-foot syndrome, neuropathy, neutropenia), without increasing treatment-related mortality.[5,7,8] Although OX-related neuropathy typically improves with discontinuation of drug, 15% of patients have at least grade 1 residual neuropathy at 4 years.[6] Despite showing a DFS benefit, the value of the weekly FLOX regimen is limited because it causes more grade 3/4 diarrhea than FOL-FOX, does not affect OS, and was associated with shorter survival after recurrence in NSABP C-07.[8] As to whether all patients with stage III disease stand to benefit from the addition of OX, guidelines suggest restricting the use of OX to patients younger than 70 years based on data suggesting that elderly patients do not benefit from the addition of OX to leucovorin infusional/bolus 5-fluorouracil (LV5FU2).[9,10]

Despite proven benefits in the metastatic setting, the addition of irinotecan (IRI) is not indicated in the adjuvant study. The results of Pan European Trial Adjuvant Colon Cancer (PETACC)-3, FNCLCC Accord02/FFCD9802, and Cancer and Leukemia Group B (CALGB) 89803 failed to show an incremental benefit from addition of IRI to standard infusional LV5FU2 or bolus FU/LV (see **Table 2**).[11–13] Combination therapy was associated with greater toxicity, and in combination with bolus FU/LV, IRI increased treatment mortality in the adjuvant setting.[12]

Targeted agents have been similarly ineffective in the adjuvant setting (**Table 3**). The addition of bevacizumab (BEV), a humanized monoclonal antibody directed against VEGF, to OX-based chemotherapy increased toxicity (eg, grade 3/4 hypertension, serious adverse events) without an improvement in DFS.[14–16] Furthermore, the results of the AVANT trial suggested a potential detrimental effect on OS with BEV in patients with stage II/III colon cancer.[14] Similarly, regardless of KRAS (Kirsten rat sarcoma viral oncogene homolog) mutational status, the addition of cetuximab, an antibody to the EGFR to mFOLFOX6 increased toxicity (particularly in older patients), without improving DFS in patients with stage III disease.[17] A trend toward improved DFS and OS was observed with cetuximab in a small subgroup of patients treated with infusional/bolus FU, LV, IRI (FOLFIRI).[18]

Stage II Colon Cancer

The optimal therapy for stage II disease remains controversial given an expected 5-year OS of 75% or greater. At a minimum, the available evidence suggests that less is more in patients without high-risk features. The results of 2 meta-analyses[19,20] suggest that nearly all of the benefit of adjuvant therapy with FP-based therapy is in patients with stage III disease. A small, but statistically significant, improvement in OS was noted in the QUASAR (Quick and Simple and Reliable) trial with adjuvant FU/LV, but the results may have been confounded because many patients were high risk by virtue of having fewer than 12 lymph nodes sampled.[21] Another meta-analysis[22] yielded similarly conflicting results, possibly stemming from inclusion of nontraditional chemotherapy regimens and lack of surgical quality control. A post hoc exploratory analysis of DFS and OS in the MOSAIC study showed that the addition of OX is also without obvious benefit (compared with FU/LV alone) in patients with stage II disease.[9] Taken together, the data suggest that less is more in patients with low-risk stage II colon cancer. The incremental benefit of adjuvant FU/LV is modest at best, and the benefits of adding OX unclear. In low-risk stage II patients, current recommendations are to use an FP alone if chemotherapy is considered.

In patients with high-risk stage II disease (defined as harboring poor prognostic features), adjuvant chemotherapy is often considered based on subset analyses,

Table 3
Results of selected phase 3 adjuvant trials with targeted agents in colon cancer

Study	Stage	Study Arms	N	Primary Endpoint	DFS (%)	OS (%)	Reference
BEV-Based							
NSABP C-08	II/III II/III	FOLFOX6+BEV FOLFOX6	2673	DFS in stage III	No change at 3 or 5 y	No change at 5 y	Allegra et al,[15,16] 2011
AVANT	II/III	FOLFOX4 BEV+FOLFOX4 BEV+XELOX	3451	DFS in stage III	No change at 4 y	BEV+FOLFOX/FOLFOX HR = 1.27; 95% CI, 1.03 to 1.57; P = .02 BEV+XELOX/FOLFOX HR = 1.15; 95% CI, 0.93 to 1.42; P = .21	de Gramont et al,[14] 2012
Cetuximab-Based							
N0147	III	FOLFOX6+cetuximab FOLFOX6	2686	DFS	No change at 3 y (regardless of KRAS status)	No change	Alberts et al,[17] 2012

Abbreviations: BEV, bevacizumab; DFS, disease-free survival; FOLFOX, infusional/bolus 5-fluorouracil, leucovorin, oxaliplatin; HR, hazard ratio; KRAS, Kirsten rat sarcoma viral oncogene homolog; OS, overall survival; XELOX, capecitabine/oxaliplatin.

suggesting a higher likelihood of recurrence in this population.[23] However, neither FLOX nor FOLFOX has been shown to be associated with improved OS over FP treatment alone in stage II patients with high-risk features.[9,10]

Ongoing studies are aimed at validating predictive markers that may be used to prospectively select the patients most likely to benefit from adjuvant therapy in stage II disease. Microsatellite instability (MSI) is a marker of more favorable outcome and may be a predictor of decreased benefit from adjuvant therapy with FP alone in stage II disease.[24–26] The available data[24,26] suggest that patients with resected MSI-high stage II colon cancers have an excellent prognosis and are unlikely to benefit from FP alone in the adjuvant setting. Several multigene assays have also been developed that may help to identify the stage II patients most likely to benefit. However, although the panels seem to have prognostic value, their predictive value in terms of response to chemotherapy remains to be established.[26]

ADJUVANT/NEOADJUVANT COMBINATION THERAPY FOR RESECTABLE RECTAL CANCER
Chemoradiation

The treatment of rectal cancer is based on the stage of the tumor, goals of care, patient preference, and the likely functional result (eg, bowel, urinary, sexual function). Patients with stage I disease are treated with surgery alone. The treatment of patients with stage II/III disease involves chemoradiation (CRT), surgery, and adjuvant chemotherapy. However, the relative value of the individual treatment components of multimodality therapy remains unclear, particularly in the context of patients experiencing a complete response to neoadjuvant therapy and in patients with T3N0 proximal rectal cancers (in whom the incremental value of radiation (RT) is uncertain).[27,28]

The usefulness of infusional 5FU as a radiosensitizer in stage II/III rectal cancer was established 20 years ago and has been shown to reduce the risk of relapse and improve OS compared with bolus 5FU/RT.[29] CAPE is noninferior to infusional FU.[30] Modern CRT is typically delivered in the neoadjuvant setting based on data suggesting improved outcomes (eg, reduction in local recurrence) compared with postoperative treatment.[31,32] However, a key limitation of neoadjuvant therapy is the risk of overtreatment, particularly because overstaging with preoperative imaging occurs.[33,34] On the other hand, roughly 20% of preoperatively staged cT3N0 tumors treated with neoadjuvant CRT are understaged (ie, positive lymph node involvement at surgery), suggesting potential value to overtreating cT3N0 disease.[35] Modern surgical techniques, such as total mesorectal excision, may reduce the incidence of a positive circumferential radial margin (an important pathologic staging parameter in rectal cancer), thus reducing the risk of local recurrence and potentially circumventing the need for RT in selected patients.[27,36]

Approximately 20% of patients treated with neoadjuvant CRT experience a pathologic complete response (pCR), a feature that portends a good prognosis.[37,38] Considerable effort has gone into enhancing the response to neoadjuvant treatment, either by adding radiosensitizers, incorporating preoperative chemotherapy or increasing the interval between completion of CRT and resection. The value of adding OX to traditional CRT has been assessed in several trials (**Table 4**).[39–42] Toxicity is increased without a reproducible increase in pCR rate. Many of the efficacy end points are not yet mature or have yielded conflicting results. Thus, the value of OX when added to concurrent RT for the treatment of rectal cancer remains controversial. Differences in trial design (including adjuvant chemotherapy, RT dose, and FP backbone) make cross-trial comparisons difficult.[43,44] In the

Table 4
Results of selected randomized trials of OX-based therapy in localized rectal cancer

Study	Study Arms	N	First End Point	DFS (%)	OS (%)	Local Recurrence (%)	pCR Rate (%)	Reference
ACCORD 12	CAPE-RT+OX/CAPE-RT (preoperative)	598	pCR	No change at 3 y	No change at 3 y	No change at 3 y	19.2/13.9 No change	Gerard et al,[42] 2012
STAR-01	FU-RT+OX/FU-RT (preoperative)	747	OS	TBD	TBD	No change at 3 y	16/16 No change	Aschele et al,[39] 2011
R-04	Continuous infusion FU-RT ± OX CAPE-RT ± OX preoperative	2407	Local recurrence	TBD	TBD	TBD	No change[a]	O'Connell et al,[41] 2014
CAO/ARO/AIO-04	CRT+OX-S-FOLFOX/CRT-S-bolus FU/LV	1265	DFS	75.9/71.2 at 3 y 68.8/64.3 at 5 y HR = 0.79, 95% CI .64-.98; $P = .030$	No change	TBD	17/13 HR = 1.40, 95% CI 1.02-1.92; $P = .038$ (exploratory)	Rodel et al,[40] 2012 Rodel et al,[43] 2014
PETACC-6	CAPE, OX, RT-S-CAPOX/CAPE, RT-S-CAPE	1094	DFS	No change at 3 y (interim)	TBD	TBD	TBD	Schmoll et al,[44] 2014

Abbreviations: CAPE, capecitabine; CAPOX, capecitabine, oxaliplatin; CI, confidence interval; CRT, chemoradiation therapy; DFS, disease-free survival; FU, 5-fluorouracil; FU/LV, bolus 5-fluorouracil, leucovorin; HR, hazard ratio; OS, overall survival; OX, oxaliplatin; pCR, pathologic complete response; RT, radiation therapy; S, surgery; TBD, to be determined.
[a] Also no change in sphincter-sparing procedures or surgical downstaging.

German CAO/ARO/AIO-04 study, improved pCR and DFS (but not OS) were observed with OX, but study patients received a more protracted schedule of infusional FU during CRT and FOLFOX instead of bolus FU/LV in the adjuvant setting. These features raise the possibility that more might not have been better had control patients received protracted FU infusion during CRT and adjuvant infusional LV5FU2.[40] Additional trials assessing the optimal treatment of localized rectal cancer are ongoing (**Table 5**).

Table 5
Selected ongoing phase 3 trials of adjuvant/neoadjuvant therapy for rectal cancer[a]

Study ID	Stage	Study Arms	Location
Role of RT			
FDRT-002	II/III	High-intensity vs low-intensity neoadjuvant CRT	China
BE-2-48	II/III	Short course RT vs conventional CRT followed by surgery	Lithuania
NL36315.042.11	T4 or N2 tumors	Short course RT followed by CAPOX × 6 vs conventional CRT	Netherlands + others
FDRT-002	II/III	Neoadjuvant FU/RT vs FOLFOX × 4 followed by FU/RT vs FOLFOX × 4 without RT	China
N1048	II/III	Neoadjuvant FOLFOX × 6 followed by selective use of CRT vs standard CRT	NCCTG, United States
CRCCZ-R01	II/III with (-) CRM by MRI	Neoadjuvant CRT followed by surgery vs surgery followed by selective use of CRT	China[b]
9100013841	III	CRT vs wide pelvic lymphadenectomy	Taiwan
4-2014-0239	II/III with (-) CRM by MRI	TME ± adjuvant FOLFOX in patient with (-) CRM	China[b]
Role of Chemotherapy			
AERO-R98	II/III	Adjuvant FU/LV vs LV5FU2+IRI	France
CAMS_rectal cancer_01	II/III	Adjuvant CRT with capecitabine vs OX plus capecitabine	China
515(A1144)/2005	II/III	Neoadjuvant RT with chronomodulated capecitabine with or without OX	Italy
PRODIGE 23	II/II	Neoadjuvant mFOLFIRINOX then CRT vs CRT alone	France
NP-113/2011	T3,4N0,1M0	Adjuvant 5FU/OX × 4 mo vs observation	Brazil
CDR0000613042	II/III	12 vs 6 cycles OxMdG or XELOX	UK
Timing of Surgery			
P 110125	II/III	Surgery after 7 vs 11 wk delay after CRT	France

Abbreviations: CAPOX, capecitabine, oxaliplatin; CRM, circumferential margin; CRT, chemoradiation; FU/LV, bolus 5-fluorouracil, leucovorin; FU, 5-fluorouracil; IRI, irinotecan; LV5FU2, infusional/bolus 5-fluorouracil, leucovorin; mFOLFIRINOX, infusional/bolus 5-fluorouracil, leucovorin, oxaliplatin, irinotecan; OX, oxaliplatin; OxMdG/FOLFOX/XELOX, infusional/bolus 5-fluorouracil, leucovorin, oxaliplatin; RT, radiation therapy; TME, total mesorectal excision.
[a] http://www.clinicaltrials.gov.
[b] Approved, not yet active.

Phase 2 studies exploring the value of IRI, EGFR inhibitors, or BEV to improve the response to neoadjuvant CRT have been performed; however, phase 3 data are not yet available.[45] Use of these agents is not recommended outside a clinical trial.

Adjuvant Chemotherapy for Rectal Cancer

The treatment of stage II/III rectal cancer typically includes adjuvant chemotherapy with FU/LV.[29,31,46] The role of adjuvant chemotherapy relative to CRT has been difficult to ascertain, although 1 meta-analysis suggested that adjuvant chemotherapy improves DFS and OS.[47] Other regimens (eg, FOLFOX, CAPOX [capecitabine/OX], and CAPE) have been used by extrapolation from colon cancer (see **Table 4**). The PETACC-6 and AIO/ARO/AI-04 trials both evaluated OX-based chemotherapy for rectal cancer, but yielded conflicting results.[43,44] Ongoing studies are designed to further optimize chemotherapy for localized rectal cancer, including addressing the potential for preoperative chemotherapy to replace the need for CRT entirely (see **Table 5**).

FIRST-LINE THERAPY FOR METASTATIC COLORECTAL CANCER
Single-Agent Chemotherapy

The treatment of metastatic colorectal cancer (mCRC) has evolved dramatically over the past 15 years (**Tables 6** and **7**). Several agents (FU/LVCAPE, OX, and IRI) are routinely used in a variety of single-agent and combination chemotherapy regimens. Infusional FU is better tolerated (less granulocytopenia, diarrhea, and mucositis) and more efficacious than bolus FU.[48] CAPE is superior to bolus FU in the first-line setting (improved RR, with less diarrhea, nausea, stomatitis, and alopecia, and fewer hospitalizations) but is associated with a higher rate of hyperbilirubinemia and hand-foot syndrome.[49,50] As in the adjuvant setting, CAPE seems to be equivalent to infusional FU in the treatment of metastatic disease.[51–53] In combination with bolus FU, the addition of LV improves OS, but use of more (eg, high-dose) LV does not seem to be superior to low-dose drug.[54,55] There is no obvious benefit to adding LV to protracted 5FU infusions.[56] Historically, patients treated with an FP alone could expect a 15% to 20% RR, median progression-free survival (PFS) 5 to 6 months and OS 10 to 14 months.[56] By themselves, OX and IRI have limited activity in the first-line setting.[57–59]

Doublet Chemotherapy

Combination therapy with an FP plus IRI or OX is associated with improved RRs, PFS, and OS compared with treatment with an FP alone, but at the expense of added toxicity (see **Tables 6** and **7**).[60] CAPOX has similar efficacy to FOLFOX and an acceptable safety profile. FOLFOX is associated with more grade 3/4 neutropenia, febrile neutropenia, and venous thromboembolic events; CAPOX is associated with more grade 3 diarrhea (19% vs 11%) and grade 3 hand-foot syndrome (6% vs 1%).[61,62] In terms of IRI-based combinations, FOLFIRI is associated with a longer PFS than irinotecan, 5-fluorouracil, and leucovorin (IFL), a less tolerable bolus regimen that is no longer used.[63] The results with CAPIRI have been mixed. Several European studies[64,65] have shown promising results and good tolerability with CAPIRI-based treatment; others[66] have been stopped prematurely because of serious toxicity concerns. The BICC-C study showed that CAPIRI was less active than FOLFIRI (PFS), and associated with more grade 3 or higher nausea, vomiting, dehydration, diarrhea, dehydration, and hand-foot syndrome.[67] CAPIRI is not a routinely recommended regimen in the United States.

Table 6
Results of selected phase 3 trials of first-line chemotherapy alone for metastatic colorectal cancer[a]

Regimen	First End Point	Study Arms	N	RR (%)	PFS	OS	Reference
FP alone	RR	Bolus FU + high-dose LV	148	21.6	39.3 wk	55 wk	Jager et al,[54] 1996
		Bolus FU + low-dose LV	143	17.5	30 wk	54 wk	de Gramont et al,[48] 1997
	OS	Bolus FU/LV	173	14.5	22 wk	56.8 wk	
		LV5FU2	175	32.6, $P = .0004$	27.6 wk, $P = .001$	62 mo	Van Cutsem et al,[50] 2004
	b	CAPE	603	26, $P = .002$	4.6 mo	12.9 mo	
		Bolus FU/LV	604	17	4.7 mo	12.8 mo	
Doublet chemotherapy	PFS	LV5FU2	210	22.3	6.2	14.7 mo	de Gramont et al,[60] 2000
		LV5FU2+OX	210	50.7, $P = .0001$	9.0, $P = .0003$	16.2 mo	
	PFS	CAPOX	242	48	7.1	16.8 mo	Porschen et al,[125] 2007
		FUFOX	234	54	8.0	18.8 mo	
	PFS	XELOX (± placebo or BEV)	1017	47	8.0	19.8 mo	Cassidy et al,[61] 2011
		FOLFOX4 (± placebo or BEV)	1017	48	8.5	19.6 mo	
	PFS	FOLFIRI	144	47.2	7.6	23.1 mo	Fuchs et al,[67] 2007
		mIFL	141	43.3	5.9; $P = .004$	17.6 mo	
		CAPIRI	145	38.6	5.8; $P = .015$	18.9 mo	
	TTP	mIFL	151	32	5.5	16.4 mo	Goldberg et al,[63] 2006
		FOLFOX	154	48, $P = .006$	9.7, $P<.0001$	19.0 mo, $P<.026$	Ashley et al,[126] 2007
		IROX	383	36.4, $P = .002$	6.7, $P<.001$	17.3 mo, $P = .001$	
	PFS	FOLFIRI→FOLFOX	109	56	8.5	21.5 mo	Tournigand, et al,[68] 2004
		FOLFOX→FOLFIRI	111	54	8.0	20.6 mo	
	RR	FOLFIRI	164[i]	31	9	14 mo	Colucci et al,[105] 2005
		FOLFOX4	172	34	10	15 mo	
Triplet chemotherapy	RR	FOLFOXIRI	122	60	9.8	22.6	Falcone et al,[92] 2007
		FOLFIRI	122	34, $P<.0001$	6.9, $P = .0006$	16.7, $P = .032$	
	OS	FOLFOXIRI	137	43	8.4	21.5	Souglakos et al,[93] 2006
		FOLFIRI	146	33.6	6.9	19.5	

Abbreviations: BEV, bevacizumab; CAPE, capecitabine; CAPIRI, capecitabine, irinotecan; CAPOX/XELOX, capecitabine/oxaliplatin; FOLFIRI, bolus and infusional 5-fluorouracil, leucovorin, irinotecan; FOLFOX, bolus and infusional 5-fluorouracil, leucovorin, oxaliplatin; FOLFOXIRI, infusional 5-fluorouracil, oxaliplatin, irinotecan, leucovorin, ± bolus 5-fluorouracil; FP, fluoropyrimidine; FU, 5-fluorouracil; FU/LV, bolus 5-fluorouracil, leucovorin; FUFOX, oxaliplatin, leucovorin, infusional 5-fluorouracil; IFL, bolus irinotecan, 5-fluorouracil, leucovorin; IROX, irinotecan, oxaliplatin; LV, leucovorin; LV5FU2, bolus and infusional 5-fluorouracil, leucovorin; OS, overall survival; OX, oxaliplatin; PFS, progression-free survival; RR, radiographic response rate.

[a] No significant change unless P value provided.
[b] Pooled data from 2 phase 3 trials.

Table 7

Incidence (%) of selected grade 3 and 4 adverse events in trials of first-line doublet chemotherapy ± biologics in metastatic colorectal cancer

Study Arms	N	Neutropenia	Febrile Neutropenia/Infection	Diarrhea	Somatitis	Neurotoxicity	Fatigue/Asthenia	Skin Toxicity (+HFS)	Hypertension	Reference
LV5FU2	210	5.3	NR/1.5	5.3	1.5	0	5	NR	NR	de Gramont et al,[60] 2000
FOLFOX	210	42a	NR/1.5	12a	6a	18a	5.6	NR	NR	
FOLFOX4	649	44a	4.8a/NR	11	2	4	9/4	1	NR	Cassidy et al,[62] 2008
CAPOX	655	7	0.9/NR	19a	1	4	6/5	6a	NR	
FOLFIRI	137	43	3.6/NR	14	NR	NR	NR	0	NR	Fuchs et al,[67] 2007
IFL	137	41	12/NR	19	NR	NR	NR	0	NR	
CAPIRI	141	32	7/NR	48a	NR	NR	NR	10a	NR	
FOLFIRI	164	10	NR	10	1	0	0	0	NR	Colucci et al,[105] 2005
FOLFOX	172	10	NR	5	1	4	0	0	NR	
FOLFIRI	602	25	NR	11	NR	NR	5	0	NR	Van Cutsem et al,[82] 2009
FOLFIRI+cetux	600	28	NR	16	NR	NR	5	20	NR	
FOLFOX	327	42	2	9	<1	16	3	2	NR	Douillard et al,[83] 2010
FOLFOX+Pmab	322	43	2	18	9	16	10	37	NR	
FOLFOX4	168	34	NR	7	1	7	3	1	NR	Bokemeyer et al,[90] 2010
FOLFOX4+cetux	170	30	NR	8	3	4	5	18	NR	
FOLFIRI-cetux	297	12.8	1.7/NR	11.5	3.7	NR	0.7/NR	17	6.4	Heinemann et al,[107] 2013
FOLFIRI-BEV	295	11.2	1/NR	13.6	4.1	NR	1.4/NR	0	6.8	
Chemo-cetux	547	NR	NR	NR	NR	12	NR	7	1	Venook et al,[91] 2014
Chemo-BEV	534	NR	NR	NR	NR	14	NR	0	7	

Abbreviations: BEV, bevacizumab; CAPIRI, capecitabine, irinotecan; CAPOX, capecitabine/oxaliplatin; cetux, cetuximab; FOLFIRI, bolus and infusional 5-fluorouracil, leucovorin, irinotecan; FOLFOX, bolus and infusional 5-fluorouracil, leucovorin, oxaliplatin; HFS, hand-foot syndrome; IFL, bolus irinotecan, 5-flurouracil, leucovorin; LV5FU2, bolus and infusional 5-fluorouracil, leucovorin; N, sample size; NR, not reported; Pmab, panitumumab.
a Statistically significant difference.

FOLFOX, FOLFIRI, and CAPOX have similar efficacy in the first-line setting.[62,68] With doublet chemotherapy, patients can expect 40% to 50% RR, median PFS 8 to 9 months, and median OS 16 to 19 months, which compares favorably with historical data with an FP alone.[60] In the absence of obvious contraindication, patients are routinely treated with at least doublet combination chemotherapy in the first-line setting. The results of a meta-analysis including more than 6000 patients suggested that the risk/benefit ratio of doublet therapy in the first-line setting is preserved in patients with performance status (PS) 2 or 1 or less, although the risks of some gastrointestinal toxicities were increased in PS 2 patients.[69]

The optimal sequence for the various doublet chemotherapy regimens remains uncertain, as is the need for up-front combination therapy in all patients. Tournigand and colleagues[68] reported that FOLFIRI and FOLFOX are equally viable options in the first-line setting (when opposite regimen used second-line). Three other studies have explored whether combination therapy up-front is essential, recognizing that improvements in OS with doublet therapy may reflect subsequent lines of therapy. In the absence of targeted therapy, there is little difference in outcome whether a patient starts with combination therapy or a less intensive regimen.[65,70,71] The French group[70] compared mLV5FU2, then FOLFOX, then FOLFIRI versus FOLFOX, then FOLFIRI in patients with unresectable mCRC. Median PFS after 2 lines of therapy was similar in the 2 groups (around 10 months) but grade 3/4 events and toxic deaths were more common in patients treated with up-front combination therapy. The CAIRO study[65] examined sequential treatment (CAPE, then IRI, then CAPOX) or combination therapy (CAPIRI, then CAPOX) in 820 patients. There was no difference in OS (16.3 months vs 17.4 months; HR = 0.92 (95% CI, 0.79–1.08; P = .3281)). Grade 3/4 toxicity was similar between groups except for more hand-foot syndrome in the sequential group. The MRC FOCUS study[71] was designed to compare (1) LV5FU2, then (2) IRI LV5FU2, then combination therapy (FOLFOX or FOLFIRI); and (3) combination therapy up-front. The median OS was similar in all groups (13.9 months in control), with the exception of patients assigned to up-front FOLFIRI (median OS 17.7; P = .01). Taken together, these data are consistent with the hypothesis that exposure to IRI OX, FP at some point in the disease course is more important than the specific sequence.[72] Although compelling, the studies on sequencing chemotherapy regimens in mCRC should be interpreted with caution in the era of targeted therapy.

Doublet Chemotherapy Regimen Plus a Vascular Endothelial Growth Factor Inhibitor

BEV has been shown to improve OS compared with chemotherapy in numerous trials in patients with mCRC (see **Table 7**; **Tables 8** and **9**). The first study was performed in patients receiving a now antiquated regimen (IFL) and was associated with a nearly 5-month improvement in OS (20.3 months vs 15.6 months; HR, 0.66; P<.001).[73] Similarly, a combined analysis of several trials showed a 3-month benefit of BEV combined with FU/LV compared with FU/LV (with or without IRI).[74]

More recent efforts have been focused on the incremental benefit of adding BEV to modern doublet regimens.[75–78] In a 1400-patient study[79] evaluating BEV in combination with OX-based chemotherapy (FOLFOX or CAPOX), BEV improved PFS by 1.4 months compared with treatment with chemotherapy alone. Combination therapy was not associated with significant improvements in OS or RR, leading many to wonder if the chemotherapy partner is an important determinant of benefit. Treatment was stopped for reasons besides cancer progression in most patients, potentially affecting survival end points, but probably not response (the overall treatment duration of BEV/placebo was only 6 months in both arms). Treatment was generally well

Table 8
Results of selected randomized trials of first-line chemotherapy + bevacizumab for metastatic colorectal cancer[a]

Regimen	First End Point	Study Arms	N	RR (%)	PFS (TTP) (mo)	OS (mo)	Reference
Doublet	OS	IFL	411	34.8	6.2	15.3	Hurwitz et al,[73] 2004
		IFL+BEV	402	44.8, P = .004	10.6, P<.001	20.6, P<.001	
	PFS	IFL+BEV	60	53.5	8.3	19.2	Fuchs et al,[77] 2008
		FOLFIRI+BEV	57	57.9	11.2	28.0, P = .037; HR = 1.79; 95% CI, 1.12 to 2.88	
	PFS	XELIRI+BEV	143	38.5	10.2	20.0	Pectasides et al,[64] 2012
		FOLFIRI+BEV	142	40.1	10.8'	25.3	
	PFS	FOLFIRI+BEV	209	53.1	11.1	22.2	Sobrero et al,[78] 2009
	PFS	FOLFOX/XELOX-Placebo	701	47	8.0	19.9	Saltz et al,[79] 2008
		FOLFOX/XELOX-BEV	699	49	9.4, P = .0023	21.3	
	AE[b]	FOLFOX/BEV	71	52	(9.9)	26.1	Hochster et al,[75] 2008
		bFOL/BEV	70	39	(8.3)	20.4	
		CAPOX/BEV	72	46	(10.3)	24.6	
Triplet therapy	PFS	FOLFIRI/BEV	256	53	9.7	25.8	Falcone et al,[94] 2013
		FOLFOXIRI/BEV	252	65, P = .006	12.2, P = .0012	31.0 (preliminary, no change)	
	R0-2 rate	FOLFOX6/BEV	39	61.5	Not mature	NR	Gruenberger et al,[96] 2013
		FOLFOXIRI/BEV	41	81.5			

Abbreviations: AE, adverse event rate; BEV, bevacizumab; bFOL, oxaliplatin, weekly bolus fluorouracil, leucovorin; CAPOX/XELOX, capecitabine/oxaliplatin; CI, confidence interval; FOLFIRI, bolus and infusional 5-fluorouracil, leucovorin, irinotecan; FOLFOX, bolus and infusional 5-fluorouracil, leucovorin, oxaliplatin; FOLFOXIRI, infusional 5-fluorouracil, oxaliplatin, irinotecan, leucovorin, ± bolus 5-fluorouracil; HR, hazard ratio; IFL, bolus irinotecan, 5-flurouracil, leucovorin; NR, not reported; OS, overall survival; PFS, progression-free survival; R0-2, resection rate; RR, radiographic response rate; TTP, time to progression; XELIRI, capecitabine, irinotecan.
[a] No significant change unless P value provided.
[b] Grade 3/4 adverse events in the first 12 wk.

Table 9
Results of phase 3 trials comparing targeted agents in combination with first-line doublet chemotherapy for metastatic colorectal cancer[a]

Regimen	First End Point	Study Arms	N	RR (%)	PFS (mo)	OS (mo)	Reference
CALGB 80405 (KRAS WT)	OS	Chemo (FOLFOX or FOLFIRI) + BEV	559	NR	10.8	29.0	Venook et al,[91] 2014
		Chemo (FOLFOX or FOLFIRI) + cetux	578	NR	10.4	29.9	
		FOLFOX + BEV	409	NR		26.9	
		FOLFOX + cetux	426	NR		30.1	
		FOLFIRI + BEV	150	NR		33.4	
		FOLFIRI + cetux	152			28.9	
FIRE-3 (KRAS WT)	RR	FOLFIRI + BEV	295	58	10.3	25.0	Heinemann et al,[107] 2013
		FOLFIRI + cetux	297	62	10.0	28.7, $P = .017$	

Abbreviations: BEV, bevacizumab; cetux, cetuximab; FOLFIRI, bolus and infusional 5-fluorouracil, leucovorin, irinotecan; FOLFOX, bolus and infusional 5-fluorouracil, leucovorin, oxaliplatin; KRAS, Kirsten rat sarcoma viral oncogene homolog; KRAS WT, KRAS wild-type; NR, not reported; OS, overall survival; PFS, progression-free survival; RR, radiographic response rate.
[a] No significant change unless P value provided.

tolerated, with only a minor increase (+5%) in grade 3/4 events with BEV; gastrointestinal symptoms (32% vs 27%), cardiac disorders (4% vs <1%), and hand-foot syndrome (7% vs 3%) were also increased. Additional BEV-related events were rare (eg, thromboembolic events, gastrointestinal bleeding or perforation, wound healing problems). BEV is also well tolerated in combination with FOLFIRI and shows added activity relative to historical controls.[77,78] A recent meta-analysis reported that the addition of BEV to chemotherapy is associated with higher treatment-related mortality, with hemorrhage, neutropenia, and gastrointestinal perforation being the most common cause of fatality.[80]

Doublet Chemotherapy Regimen Plus Epidermal Growth Factor Receptor Inhibitor

Several studies have reported the value of an EGFR inhibitor in combination with first-line doublet chemotherapy in KRAS wild-type (WT) tumors (see **Tables 7** and **9**; **Table 10**).[81–83] Typical side effects of antibody treatment include skin toxicity, hypersensitivity reactions, diarrhea, hypokalemia, hypomagnesemia, and fatigue. The severity of the rash seems to be predictive of response to therapy, suggesting that more may be better in patients without a significant rash.[84] The presence of a mutation in codon 12 or 13 of exon 2 of the KRAS gene (present in 40% patients with mCRC) predicts for lack of benefit from EGFR antibodies; some studies even suggest a detrimental effect on outcome when patients with KRAS mutant tumors are treated.[85] In addition, emerging data have shown that NRAS mutations and KRAS mutations outside exon 2 (encompassed by expanded RAS testing) also have predictive value.[86] BRAF V600E mutations occur in 5% to 9% of patients with mCRC. Although it indicates a poor prognosis, the predictive value of the BRAF V600E mutation is uncertain. Studies have suggested that the mutation predicts for resistance to EGFR inhibitors in the salvage setting, but not in the first-line setting.[87]

The optimal chemotherapy partner for EGFR inhibitors in mCRC is controversial, stemming from conflicting data from studies using OX-based or CAPE-based

Table 10
Results of selected randomized trials of first-line chemotherapy + EGFR inhibitor for metastatic colorectal cancer[a]

Regimen	First End Point	Study Arms	N	RR (%)	PFS (TTP) (mo)	OS (mo)	Reference
Doublet Chemotherapy							
CRYSTAL	PFS	FOLFIRI	599	38.7	8.0	18.6	Van Cutsem et al,[82] 2009
		FOLFIRI + cetux	599	46.9, P = .004	8.9, P = .048	19.9	
CRYSTAL		FOLFIRI (WT-KRAS)	176	43.2	8.7	21	
		FOLFIRI-cetux (WT-RAS)	172	59.3, P = .03	9.9	24.9	
		FOLFIRI (MT-KRAS)	87	36.2	8.1	17.7	
		FOLFIRI-cetux (MT-KRAS)	105	40.2	7.6	17.5	
PRIME	PFS	FOLFOX4 (WT-KRAS)	331	48	8.6	19.7	Douillard et al,[83] 2010
		FOLFOX4 + Pmab (WT-KRAS)	325	57, P = .02	10, P = .01	23.9	
		FOLFOX4 (MT-KRAS)	219	41	9.2	19.2	
		FOLFOX4 + Pmab (MT-KRAS)	221	40	7.4, P = .02	15.5	
OPUS	RR	FOLFOX4	168	36	7.2	18.0	Bokemeyer et al,[90] 2011
		FOLFOX4 + cetux	169	46	7.2	18.3	
OPUS		FOLFOX4 (WT-KRAS)	97	34	7.2	18.5	
		FOLFOX4 + cetux (WT-KRAS)	82	57, P = .0027	8.3, P = .0064	22.8	
		FOLFOX4 (MT-KRAS)	59	53	8.6	17.5	
		FOLFOX4 + cetux (MT-KRAS)	77	34, P = .029	5.5, P = .015	13.4	
MRC COIN (KRAS WT subtype)	OS	OX-based chemo (WT-KRAS)	367	57	8.6	17.9	Maughan et al,[89] 2011
		OX-based chemo + cetux (WT-KRAS)	362	64, P = .049	8.6	17.0	
NORDIC VII (KRAS WT subset)	PFS	FLOX	97	47	8.7	22.0	Tveit, et al,[88] 2012
		Cetux + FLOX	97	46	7.9	20.1	
		Cetux + intermittent FLOX	109	51	7.5	21.4	
Triplet Chemotherapy							
RAS WT/BRAF WT		FOLFOXIRI/Pmab	37	89	11.3	NR	Fornaro et al,[98] 2013
KRAS WT		FOLFOXIRI/cetux	20	75	16	33	Folprecht et al,[97] 2014

Abbreviations: cetux, cetuximab; FLOX, oxaliplatin, folus 5-fluorouracil, leucovorin; FOLFIRI, bolus and infusional 5-fluorouracil, leucovorin, irinotecan; FOLFOX, bolus and infusional 5-fluorouracil, leucovorin, oxaliplatin; FOLFOXIRI, infusional 5-fluorouracil, oxaliplatin, irinotecan, leucovorin, ± bolus 5-fluorouracil; KRAS, Kirsten rat sarcoma viral oncogene homolog; MT, mutant; NR, not reported; OS, overall survival; OX, oxaliplatin; PFS, progression-free survival; Pmab, panitumumab; RR, radiographic response rate; TTP, time to progression; WT, wild-type.
[a] No significant change unless P value provided.

regimens. Despite the encouraging results noted in the OPUS study with FOLFOX/cetuximab, neither the COIN study (OX-based chemotherapy ± cetuximab) nor the NORDIC VII studies (FLOX/cetuximab) reached their primary end point, even when the analysis was limited to KRAS WT tumors.[88–90] Most of the patients in COIN were treated with a CAPE backbone, leading some to wonder if CAPE is a suboptimal partner for cetuximab. Regardless, some of these concerns were alleviated with the release of the Intergroup 80,405 results suggesting that chemotherapy/cetuximab and chemotherapy/BEV are comparable first-line treatments for patients with KRAS WT mCRC.[91] The median OS was excellent in both groups (approximately 29 months). Most patients in this trial were treated with FOLFOX, and a smaller group received FOLFIRI; CAPE-based therapy was not allowed.

Triplet Chemotherapy

The role of triplet therapy (eg, FOLFIRINOX) remains controversial given concerns about added toxicity, downstream treatment options, and the value of the established incremental benefit (see **Table 6**; **Table 11**). Falcone and colleagues[92] reported on 244 fit patients with mCRC treated in the first-line setting. Treatment with infusional 5FU, OX, IRI, LV, ± bolus 5FU (FOLFOXIRI) was associated with an increase in grade 2/3 neurotoxicity (0% vs 19%; $P<.001$) and grade 3/4 neutropenia (28% vs 50%; $P<.001$) compared with FOLFIRI alone; however, there was no difference in the rates of febrile neutropenia (3% vs 5%) and 60-day mortality (1.6%). RR by independent review was significantly increased with triplet therapy (34% vs 66%; $P = .0002$), as was median PFS (6.9 vs 9.8 months; HR, 0.63; $P = .0006$) and median OS (16.7 vs 22.6 months; HR, 0.70; $P = .032$). Although not specifically designed to explore resectability, R0 secondary resection rate of metastases was greater in the FOLFOXIRI arm (6% vs 15%; $P = .033$, among all patients; and 12% vs 36%; $P = .017$ among patients with liver-only disease). In a cautionary note, a parallel study (which included bolus FU) confirmed increased toxicity but failed to show a difference in RR, PFS, or OS with FOLFOXIRI compared with FOLFIRI.[93]

TRIPLET CHEMOTHERAPY PLUS BEVACIZUMAB

In the TRIBE study, patients receiving first-line triplet chemotherapy plus BEV reported improved PFS (12.2 vs 9.7 mo, $P = .0012$) and RR (65% vs 53%, $P = .006$) compared with FOLFIRI/BEV.[94] Diarrhea, stomatitis, neutropenia, and neuropathy were also significantly increased (see **Tables 8** and **11**). In a subgroup analysis, patients with previous adjuvant therapy did not seem to benefit from intensive therapy.[92] In contrast, the benefit of FOLFOXIRI/BEV was independent of BRAF mutational status (HR 0.55 in favor of triplet therapy over FOLFIRI in 28 patients with tumors harboring BRAF mutation).[95] This finding warrants further study, because patients with tumors harboring this mutation have a particularly poor prognosis and can expect a median OS with doublet chemotherapy (9–14 months) that is approximately half that of patients with tumors that are WT for BRAF.[95] The R0 resection rate (a secondary end point) was similar in both groups. In contrast, an improved R0 resection rate (49% vs 23%, $P = .017$) was observed in a small randomized phase 2 trial of FOLFOX/BEV versus FOLFOXIRI/BEV designed to assess resection rate.[96] Although intriguing, the results need to be confirmed in other studies, particularly because patient selection seems to be critically important for FOLFOXIRI-based regimens.

Table 11
Incidence (%) of selected grade 3 and 4 adverse events in selected trials of triplet chemotherapy or dual biologics for previously untreated metastatic colorectal cancer

Study Arms	N	Neutropenia	Febrile Neutropenia/Infection	Diarrhea	Somatitis	Neurotoxicity	Fatigue/Asthenia	Skin Toxicity	Hypertension	Reference
FOLFIRI	122	28	3/NR	11	3	0	3	NR	NR	Falcone, et al,[92] 2007
FOLFOXIRI	122	50[a]	5/NR	20	5	2[a]	6	NR	NR	
FOLFIRI	147	28	4/NR	11	4	0	5	3	NR	Souglakos et al,[93] 2006
FOLFOXIRI	138	35	7/NR	28[a]	5	6[a]	5.6	4	NR	
CAPOX/BEV	366	NR	NR/6.8	19	NR	10.4	13	20.8	14.8[a]	Tol et al,[100] 2009
CAPOX/BEV/cetux	366	NR	NR/6.0	26[a]	NR	7.7	15	39.1[a]	9.3	
Pmab+BEV +OX-CT	246	24	NR/18	24[a]	NR	4	NR	36[a]	4	Hecht et al,[101] 2008
BEV+OX-CT	221	24	NR/10	13	NR	7	NR	1	5	
Pmab+BEV +IRI-CT	54	17	NR/14	28[a]	NR	NR	NR	38[a]	2	Hecht et al,[101] 2008
BEV+IRI-CT	44	21	NR/9	9	NR	NR	NR	3	3	
FOLFIRI/BEV	256	20	6/NR	11	4	0	NR	NR	2	Falcone, et al,[94] 2013
FOLFOXIRI/BEV	252	50[a]	9/NR	19[a]	9[a]	5[a]	NR	NR	5	
FOLFOX/BEV	39	35	8/NR	14	NR	NR	NR	NR	NR	Gruenberger et al,[96] 2013
FOLFOXIRI/BEV	41	48	13/NR	28	NR	NR	NR	NR	NR	
FOLFOXIRI/cetux	20	40	NR/NR	25	0	NR	0	15	NR	Folprecht et al,[97] 2014
FOLFOXIRI/Pmab	37	48	5/NR	35	12	8	27	14	NR	Fornaro, et al,[98] 2013

Abbreviations: BEV, bevacizumab; CAPOX, capecitabine/oxaliplatin; cetux, cetuximab; FOLFIRI, bolus and infusional 5-fluorouracil, leucovorin, irinotecan; FOLFOX, bolus and infusional 5-fluorouracil, leucovorin, oxaliplatin; FOLFOXIRI, infusional 5-fluorouracil, oxaliplatin, irinotecan, leucovorin, ± bolus 5-fluorouracil; IRI-CT, irinotecan-based chemotherapy; NR, not reported; OX-CT, oxaliplatin-based chemotherapy; Pmab, panitumumab.
[a] Significant difference.

TRIPLET CHEMOTHERAPY PLUS AN EPIDERMAL GROWTH FACTOR RECEPTOR INHIBITOR

Recently, investigators explored the safety of adding cetuximab to FOLFOXIRI triplet therapy in PS 0-1 patients (KRAS status not assessed).[97] Cetuximab/FOLFOXIRI was feasible but required a reduced dose of IRI relative to FOLFOXIRI alone (see **Table 10**).[92] The most common grade 3 or higher toxicities were neutropenia (40%), diarrhea (25%), and acnelike rash (15%) (see **Table 11**). The preliminary efficacy appeared promising, with an overall RR 75% (all cohorts combined), median PFS 16.0 months (95% CI, 12.6–19.4), and median OS 33 months (95% CI, 26.2–39.8). The median time to maximal response was 3 months (95% CI, 2.2–3.7), suggesting potential value in the neoadjuvant setting. Seventy-five percent of patients had ECOG PS 0, and thus, the safety of cetuximab/FOLFOXIRI in patients with impaired PS is unknown. The usefulness of cetuximab/FOLFOXIRI in patients with KRAS WT unresectable liver-only mCRC is under study in an ongoing randomized phase 2 trial.

Preliminary results with FOLFOXIRI/panitumumab have yielded similarly impressive results (see **Tables 10** and **11**). Fornaro and colleagues[98] reported an RR 89% and median PFS 11.3 months (95% CI, 9.7–12.9 months) in 37 patients with unresectable KRAS, NRAS, HRAS, and BRAF WT mCRC and ECOG PS 0/1. A modified FOLFOXIRI regimen was used (decreased 5FU and IRI dose) for a maximum of 12 cycles (after which patients received panitumumab ± FU/LV). The most common grade 3 to 4 adverse events during induction treatment were neutropenia (48%; febrile neutropenia in 5%), diarrhea (35%), asthenia (27%), stomatitis (14%), and skin toxic effect (14%). One treatment-related death was reported. Most (76%) patients had ECOG PS 0. Future trials are aimed at validating the initial findings with FOLFOXIRI-based treatment, identifying the patients most likely to benefit (ie, candidates with borderline resectable disease), and exploring the role of maintenance therapy after induction therapy in molecularly selected patients.[98]

Double Targeted Agents Plus Chemotherapy

Several studies have shown that more is not better when dual biologics are added to doublet chemotherapy in the first-line setting (see **Table 11**; **Table 12**).[99,100] The results of CAIRO-2 showed that adding cetuximab to first-line CAPOX/BEV resulted in significantly shorter PFS and reduced quality of life. The detrimental effect was particularly pronounced in patients with KRAS mutant tumors treated with cetuximab, but a benefit from dual biologics could not be shown even when the analysis was restricted to KRAS WT patients. Hecht and colleagues[101] reported on results with chemotherapy/BEV with or without panitumumab (PACCE trial). Patients were enrolled to distinct cohorts depending on choice of chemotherapy backbone (IRI based or OX based). Panitumumab was discontinued in both cohorts after an interim analysis showed decreased PFS and increased toxicity (skin-related toxicities, diarrhea, dehydration, hypomagnesemia, infections, and pulmonary embolism) in the panitumumab-containing arms (this trend persisted even when analyzed according to KRAS mutational status). The reasons underlying these findings are unknown, particularly given the encouraging preliminary findings in refractory disease.[76,102,103] Worse outcomes in dual-antibody–treated patients may stem from reduced dose intensity (secondary to dose delays and modifications related to excessive toxicity), a pharmacokinetic interaction, or differences in subsequent therapy. Regardless, the findings do not support the use of dual biologics with either IRI-based or OX-based first-line chemotherapy.

Table 12
Results of randomized phase 3 trials of first-line doublet chemotherapy + VEGF inhibitor and EGFR inhibitor in metastatic colorectal cancer

First End Point	Study Arms	N	RR (%) (change)	PFS (12 mo PFS)	OS (mo)	Reference
PFS	FOLFOX/BEV	124	52	(45%)	21	Saltz et al,[99] 2012
	FU/LV/BEV/cetux	123	41	(32%)	19.5	
PFS	CAPOX/BEV	378	50	10.7 mo	20.3	Tol et al,[100] 2009
	CAPOX/BEV/cetux	377	52.7	9.4 mo	19.4	
				$P = .01$		
PFS	Pmab+BEV +OX-CT	246	46	10.0 mo	19.4	Hecht et al,[101] 2009
	BEV+OX-CT	221	48	11.4 mo (HR = 1.44; 95%	24.5 (HR = 1.43;	
				CI, 1.13 to 1.85; $P = .004$)	95% CI, 1.11–1.83)	
PFS	Pmab+BEV +IRI-CT	54	43	10.1 mo	20.7	Hecht et al,[101] 2009
	BEV+IRI-CT	44	40	11.7 mo	20.5	

Abbreviations: BEV, bevacizumab; CAPOX, capecitabine/oxaliplatin; cetux, cetuximab; FOLFOX, bolus and infusional 5-fluorouracil, leucovorin, oxaliplatin; FU/LV, bolus 5-fluorouracil, leucovorin; IRI-CT, irinotecan-based chemotherapy; OS, overall survival; OX-CT, oxaliplatin-based chemotherapy; PFS, progression-free survival; Pmab, panitumumab; RR, radiographic response rate.

Choice of Regimen in the Era of Targeted Agents

Given all of the options, the choice of regimen is driven by several factors, including tumor genotype, previous therapy, comorbidities (eg, residual neuropathy or early relapse after adjuvant FOLFOX), PS, personal preference, and goals of therapy (eg, candidate for potentially curative resection vs palliative therapy). For example, FOLFOX is associated with more neuropathy and thrombocytopenia; FOLFIRI with more alopecia and gastrointestinal toxicity. Furthermore, IRI should be used with caution in patients with hyperbilirubinemia (UGT1A1*28 polymorphism or other cause),[104] and CAPE-based therapy must be used with care in patients with renal dysfunction.[105] Patients with recent or ongoing cardiac ischemia, uncontrolled hypertension, bowel obstruction, or nonhealing wound should not be treated with BEV.[106] EGFR inhibitors are contraindicated in the setting of a KRAS or NRAS mutation.[86]

Although not designed to look at sequence specifically (ie, only first-line treatment was specified), 2 recent studies explored choice of targeted agent in first-line treatment (see **Tables 7** and **9**). Neither study met its primary end point; however, Intergroup 80,405 reported that patients with KRAS WT tumors can expect similar outcomes (median OS, 29.0 vs 29.9 months; PFS, 10.4 vs 10.8 months) when treated with chemotherapy (FOLFOX or FOLFIRI) plus either BEV or cetuximab.[91] The toxicity profiles were predictable, global quality of life was unchanged, and on-study mortality was similar in both arms (2.7% with BEV, 2.1% with cetuximab). Detailed subset and biomarker analyses (eg, expanded RAS) are ongoing. Detailed information on dose intensity and time to treatment failure has not been reported. In FIRE-3, cetuximab/FOLFIRI did not improve RR or PFS compared with FOLFIRI/BEV in KRAS WT patients, but was associated with improved OS (28.8 vs 25 months; HR, 0.77; $P = .016$; 95% CI, 0.62–0.95).[107] The reason underlying this finding is not readily apparent, but interpretation of the result is confounded because the details of subsequent therapy (including maintenance therapy) were not provided. Taken together, FIRE-3 and Intergroup 80,405 suggest that patients have several treatment options in the first-line setting and that additional studies are required to identify if there are particular subgroups of patients who stand to benefit from 1 antibody or 1 chemotherapy regimen upfront. The studies also underscore the importance of accounting for subsequent lines of when assessing the efficacy of first-line treatment.

Previous studies with chemotherapy alone have suggested that exposure to all agents (FP, OX, and IRI) in any order may be more important than the specific sequence in which they are delivered.[72] Whether or not this holds true in the context of the era of targeted agents and molecular stratification remains unclear. Combination therapy may improve RR and delay PFS, but intensive therapy may not be essential for all patients (particularly in frail patients in whom one is concerned about tolerability, or in patients in whom metastasectomy is not likely to ever be feasible). In contrast, fit patients with tumors harboring BRAF V600E mutations or borderline resectable disease may be especially good candidates for intensive (ie, triplet) therapy. Several ongoing trials are designed to address the need for combination therapy up-front (**Table 13**).

First-Line Chemotherapy for Liver-Only Metastases

Resection cures approximately 30% of patients with liver-only mCRC. Although only 20% of patients are resectable up-front, approximately 10% of patients become resectable after doublet chemotherapy, with a subgroup having long-term survival.[108] There is significant interest in developing regimens that improve resectability. To this end, more may be better in the neoadjuvant setting, and the associated increase in

Table 13
Selected ongoing randomized trials of first-line therapy for metastatic colorectal cancer[a]

Study ID	Study Arms	Location
FFCD 2000–05	First-line LV5FU2, second-line mFOLFOX6, 3rd line FOLFIRI vs first-line mFOLFOX6, second-line FOLFIRI, third-line infusional FU or CAPE	EORTC, Europe
ML22011	CAPE/BEV followed by CAPIRI vs CAPIRI/BEV	Germany
CDR0000692257	CAPE/FU plus BEV vs mFOLFOX7/XELOX plus BEV in elderly patients ($\geq$70 y)	NCCTG, US
TTD-12-01	FOLFOX/BEV vs FOLFOXIRI/BEV in patients with $\geq$3 CTC	Spain
STX0112	mFOLFOX6 $\pm$ SIR spheres in patients with liver metastases	International
IRST153.01	First-line: FOLFOX/FOLFIRI $\pm$ BEV (any KRAS) Second-line study (KRAS WT only): FOLFOX/FOLFIRI $\pm$ cetux if previous BEV or FOLFOX/FOLFIRI + BEV $\pm$ cetux (no previous BEV)	Italy
STRATEGIC-1 C12- 2	FOLFIRI/cetux followed by OX-based + BEV vs OPTIMOX/BEV followed by IRI-based/BEV, followed by anti-EGFR Ab $\pm$ chemotherapy (WT-RAS patient)	GERCOR, France
CAIRO5[b]	Patients with unresectable liver-only metastases: RAS mutant: FOLFOX/FOLFIRI plus BEV vs FOLFOXIRI plus BEV RAS WT: FOLFOX/FOLFIRI plus BEV vs FOLFOX/FOLFIRI plus Pmab	Netherlands
CELIM2	Patients with unresectable liver-only metastases: Cetux/FOLFOXIRI vs cetux/FOLFIRI in patients with KRAS/BRAF WT tumors BEV/FOLFOXIRI vs BEV/FOLFIRI in KRAS mutant tumors	Germany

Abbreviations: BEV, bevacizumab; CAPE, capecitabine; CAPIRI, capecitabine, irinotecan; cetux, cetuximab; CTC, circulating tumor cells; FOLFIRI, infusional/bolus fluorouracil, leucovorin, irinotecan; FOLFOX, infusional/bolus 5-fluorouracil, leucovorin, oxaliplatin; FOLFOXIRI, bolus and infusional 5-fluorouracil, leucovorin, oxaliplatin, irinotecan; FU, 5-fluorouracil; IRI, irinotecan; KRAS, Kirsten rat sarcoma viral oncogene homolog; LV5FU2, infusional/bolus 5-fluorouracil, leucovorin; OX, oxaliplatin; Pmab, panitumumab; RAS, expanded RAS; SIR, selective internal radiation; WT, wild-type.
[a] http://www.clinicaltrials.gov.
[b] Approved, not yet active.

toxicity might be worth the risk if the R0 resection rate is increased. Regimens that induce a rapid response are particularly appealing, given concerns about hepatotoxicity with protracted chemotherapy.[109] FOLFOXIRI has been compared with FOLFIRI in 2 trials in patients with unresectable mCRC.[92,93] The R0 resection rate was higher in patients receiving FOLFOXIRI in both studies (6% vs 15%, P = .033; 4% vs 10%, P = .08); in the GONO (Gruppo Oncologico Nord Ovest) trial the 5-year survival was also increased (15% vs 8%) with FOLFOXIRI.[92]

Use of BEV-based regimens needs to be considered carefully given the need to hold BEV for at least 6 weeks before surgery. The value of neoadjuvant BEV is particularly questionable in combination with FOLFOX/XELOX, because BEV does not improve RR in combination with these regimens.[79] EGFR antibodies are an appealing alternative in patients with RAS WT tumors, because they can be given up until surgery and, in combination with chemotherapy, increase RR over chemotherapy alone.[110,111] In a randomized trial of FOLFOX/FOLFIRI $\pm$ cetuximab in patients with unresectable liver metastases, conversion to resectability was increased with cetuximab (29% vs 13%), as was R0 resection rate (25.7% vs 7.4%, P<.01).[111] A recent meta-analysis of 4 studies[112] found that the addition of cetuximab improved R0 resection rate (18% vs 11%, P = .04), but not OS. Whether the toxicity of these regimens (particularly, in combination with FOLFOXIRI) is justified in the neoadjuvant setting is unclear and warrants further study. Furthermore, enthusiasm for EGFR inhibitor–based perioperative therapy is tempered because the New-EPOC study (perioperative chemotherapy ± cetuximab in patients with KRAS WT tumors) was stopped prematurely after finding that PFS was significantly reduced in the cetuximab-containing arm (14.8 vs 24.2 months, P<.048). Additional trials are under way to further investigate the optimal strategy for improving resectability and long-term outcomes in patients with mCRC (see **Table 10**).

In addition to improving resectability, chemotherapy has the potential to improve long-term outcomes when delivered in the adjuvant setting. A pooled analysis of more than 600 patients enrolled in 3 trials of surgery alone or with systemic chemotherapy showed that chemotherapy improved PFS (pooled HR, 0.75; CI, 0.62–0.91; P = .003) and DFS (pooled HR, 0.71; CI, 0.58–0.88; P = .001), but not OS (pooled HR, 0.74; CI, 0.53–1.05; P = .088).[113] As a result, providers often treat patients with resectable disease with a total of 6 months of perioperative chemotherapy, the choice of which is based on previous treatment, required depth of response, and safety/toxicity issues.[114]

Maintenance Therapy and Drug Holidays

Faced with more effective, but more toxic, combination treatment regimens for mCRC, our basic treatment paradigm has shifted for patients with unresectable disease. Historically focused on continuous treatment until intolerable toxicity or disease progression, there is an increasing acceptance that continuous therapy may not be feasible or necessary in mCRC.[115] The optimal type/duration of maintenance therapy remains controversial, but in the setting of OX-based treatment, many advocate for discontinuing OX after 3 to 6 months of therapy or sooner for unacceptable neurotoxicity (maintaining other drugs for ≥6 months, and restarting OX at progression if tolerated, see NCCN.org).[115] The basis for this approach stems from the observation that intermittent OX reduces neurotoxicity in patients receiving FOLFOX (eg, stop-and-go, OPTIMOX strategy). However, the merits of a complete drug holiday remain uncertain. Limited data suggest that maintenance FP improves disease control (13.1 months vs 9.2 months, P = .046) without improving OS (23.8 vs 19.5 mo, P = .42) compared with an observation in patients with stable disease or better on FOLFOX.[116] In patients receiving BEV plus OX-based chemotherapy first line, the bulk of the data suggest that maintenance BEV/FP improves disease control relative to observation or BEV alone but is not associated with a consistent OS benefit.[117–119] There are no randomized data to guide maintenance therapy in the context of panitumumab-based or cetuximab-based regimens.

Breaks from continuous combination therapy (before disease progression) occur in the setting of IRI-based chemotherapy as well. In FIRE-3, patients in both arms (FOLFIRI/BEV or FOLFIRI/cetuximab) received protocol-defined therapy for only about 5 months, despite having a median PFS of 10 months in both groups.[107] Similarly, most patients in Intergroup 80,405 went off study for reasons besides disease progression.[91] Although minimal information was provided about subsequent treatment in either study, it is likely that patients went off protocol-specified therapy to pursue a drug holiday or a switch to maintenance therapy before experiencing disease progression. FOLFOXIRI-based induction chemotherapy has been capped at 12 cycles of therapy in recent trials.[92,94] Ongoing trials continue to explore the concepts of induction and maintenance therapy in mCRC (**Table 14**).

Table 14			
Selected ongoing phase 3 trials exploring maintenance therapy for metastatic colorectal cancer[a]			
Study ID	First End Point	Study Arms	Location
AERO-MC04	PFS	Maintenance capecitabine vs observation in patients with responding or SD after $\geq$6 cycles of therapy	France
2010-02-047	PFS	CAPOX × 8 followed by capecitabine maintenance vs BSC	Korea
MGN1703-C06[b]	OS	MGN1703 vs placebo in patients with CR/PR after 12–30 wk of first-line chemotherapy	UK
The SIR step trial	TTP-1	SIR spheres plus LV5FU2 vs LV5FU2 alone after 3 mo of induction chemotherapy	Belgium

Abbreviations: BSC, best supportive care; CAPOX, capecitabine/oxaliplatin; CR, complete response; LV5FU2, infusional/bolus 5-fluorouracil, leucovorin; OS, overall survival; PFS, progression-free survival; PR, partial response; SD, stable disease; SIR, selective internal radiation; TTP-1, time to first progression.
[a] http://www.clinicaltrials.gov.
[b] Approved, not yet active.

SUBSEQUENT LINES OF THERAPY

An expanding body of evidence suggests that there is value in additional treatment after progression on first-line therapy in mCRC.[120,121] A range of treatment options exists, the precise sequence of which tends to be driven by choice of first-line regimen, use of maintenance strategy or drug holiday, PS, patient/provider preference, and comorbidities. Furthermore, the distinction between lines of therapy can be blurred.[114] Patients with progression on maintenance therapy or on a drug holiday may simply restart their most recent combination regimen. In contrast, residual toxicity (eg, neuropathy) may mandate switching to a new regimen in a patient previously treated with OX (often continuing the same FP backbone). A variety of sequences incorporating FP, OX, IRI, panitumumab/cetuximab, or BEV across several lines of therapy are routinely used and hinge on choice of first-line therapy. In addition, aflibercept (in combination with FOLFIRI) and regorafenib (as a single agent) are specifically approved for refractory disease and offer a modest (1.4 months) survival benefit (as does continued BEV in the second line after use in the first-line setting).[122–124] The incremental benefit of each subsequent line of therapy is modest, but when taken together, the effects are clinically meaningful. This potential impact of maintenance and salvage therapy was exemplified by the results of the recent FIRE-3, TRIBE, and Intergroup 80,405 studies, in which excellent median OS (25–30 months) was observed in all treatment groups, and median PFS and duration of first-line therapy were exceeded.[91,94,107]

SUMMARY

The treatment of colorectal cancer has steadily changed over the past 15 years in the face of an evolving landscape of approved agents for the disease. The availability of new chemotherapeutic agents (OX, IRI, CAPE) as well as VEGF and EGFR inhibitors has translated into improved outcomes. However, although more almost always means more toxicity (and cost), more is not always better in terms of efficacy and, in some cases, leads to worse outcomes. Several key lessons have emerged that have important implications for selection, treatment, and care of patients with colorectal cancer.

In the adjuvant setting, more is better for patients younger than 70 years with stage III colon cancer, in whom the addition of OX improves outcomes compared with treatment with an FP alone (at the expense of nonlethal toxicity). The optimal duration of treatment is unclear but is no longer than 6 months. The treatment of stage II colon cancer disease remains controversial. If anything, less may be more, particularly in the setting of MSI-H tumors. Furthermore, more is not better in the context of using IRI or targeted agents in the treatment of localized colon cancer, a finding that may reflect basic differences in the biological properties of micrometastases compared with established metastatic deposits.

Ongoing studies in rectal cancer are largely focused on exploring whether less is more (eg, the value of short course RT, the value of watch and wait in the setting of a clinical complete response, and the potential merit of eliminating CRT in some patients receiving neoadjuvant chemotherapy). Advances in molecular markers and preoperative imaging should further refine our ability to individualize therapy for patients with rectal cancer, thus minimizing the potential for both overtreatment and undertreatment.

In mCRC, the optimal sequence of treatment remains ill defined. Choice of therapy is governed by several factors, including previous therapy, comorbidities, goals of therapy, tumor mutational status, and personal preference. Future studies should further allow us to optimize therapy (eg, sequence, duration, choice of regimen), particularly as our ability to stratify colorectal cancer into discrete molecular subtypes matures. It is hoped that the small incremental benefits observed with individual lines of therapy will be enhanced by better patient selection, thus improving the cost-effectiveness of our therapies (ie, avoiding unnecessary toxicity in patients who are unlikely to benefit and accepting significant side effects in the patients who stand to benefit the most from combination therapy).

REFERENCES

1. Saltz L. Adjuvant therapy for colon cancer. Surg Oncol Clin North Am 2010;19: 819–27.
2. Twelves C, Wong A, Nowacki M, et al. Capecitabine as adjuvant treatment for stage III colon cancer. N Engl J Med 2005;352:2696–704.
3. Des Guetz G, Uzzan B, Morere J, et al. Duration of adjuvant chemotherapy for patients with non-metastatic colorectal cancer. Cochrane Database Syst Rev 2010;(1):CD007046.
4. Andre T, Iveson T, Labianca R, et al. The IDEA (International Duration Evaluation of Adjuvant Chemotherapy) collaboration: prospective combined analysis of phase III trials investigating duration of adjuvant therapy with the FOLFOX (FOLFOX4 or mFOLFOX6) or XELOX (3 versus 6 months) regimen for patients with stage III colon cancer: Trial Design and current status. Curr Colorectal Cancer Rep 2013;9:261–9.
5. Andre T, Boni C, Mounedji-Boudiaf L, et al. Oxaliplatin, fluorouracil and leucovorin as adjuvant treatment for colon cancer. N Engl J Med 2004;352: 2696–704.
6. Andre T, Boni C, Navarro M, et al. Improved overall survival with oxaliplatin, fluorouracil, and leucovorin as adjuvant treatment in stage II or III colon cancer in the MOSAIC trial. J Clin Oncol 2009;27:3109–16.
7. Haller D, Tabernero J, Maroun J, et al. Capecitabine plus oxaliplatin compared with fluorouracil and folinic acid as adjuvant therapy for stage III colon cancer. J Clin Oncol 2011;29:1465–71.

8. Kuebler J, Wieand H, O'Connell J, et al. Oxaliplatin combined with weekly bolus fluorouracil and leucovorin as surgical adjuvant therapy for stage II and III colon cancer: results from NSABP C-07. J Clin Oncol 2007;25:2198–204.

9. Tournigand C, Andre T, Bonnetain F, et al. Adjuvant therapy with fluorouracil and oxaliplatin in stage II and elderly patients (between the ages of 70 and 75) with colon cancer: subgroup analyses of the Multicenter International Study of Oxaliplatin, Fluorouracil, and Leucovorin in the Adjuvant Treatment of Colon Cancer trial. J Clin Oncol 2012;30:3353–60.

10. Yothers G, O'Connell J, Allegra C. Oxaliplatin as adjuvant therapy for colon cancer: updated results of NSABP C-07 trial, including survival and subset analyses. J Clin Oncol 2011;29:3768–74.

11. Ychou M, Raoul J, Douillard J, et al. A phase III randomised trial of LV5FU2+irinotecan versus LV5FU2 alone in adjuvant high-risk colon cancer (FNCLCC Accord02/FFCD9802). Ann Oncol 2009;20:674–80.

12. Saltz L, Niedzwiecki D, Hollis D, et al. Irinotecan fluorouracil plus leucovorin is not superior to fluorouracil plus leucovorin alone as adjuvant treatment for stage III colon cancer: results of CALGB 89803. J Clin Oncol 2007;25:3456–61.

13. Van Cutsem E, Labianca R, Bodoky G, et al. Randomized phase III trial comparing biweekly infusional fluorouracil/leucovorin alone or with irinotecan in the adjuvant treatment of stage III colon cancer: PETACC-3. J Clin Oncol 2009;27:3117–25.

14. de Gramont A, Van Cutsem E, Schmoll H, et al. Bevacizumab plus oxaliplatin-based chemotherapy as adjuvant treatment for colon cancer (AVANT): a phase 3 randomized controlled trial. Lancet Oncol 2012;13:1225–33.

15. Allegra C, Yothers G, O'Connell J, et al. Phase III trial assessing bevacizumab in stages II and III carcinoma of the colon: results of NSABP protocol C-08. J Clin Oncol 2011;29:11–6.

16. Allegra C, Yothers G, O'Connell J, et al. Bevacizumab in stage II-III colon cancer: 5-year update of the National Surgical Adjuvant Breast and Bowel Project C-08 trial. J Clin Oncol 2013;31:359–64.

17. Alberts S, Sargent D, Nair S, et al. Effect of oxaliplatin, fluorouracil, and leucovorin with or without cetuximab on survival among patients with resected stage III colon cancer: a randomized trial. JAMA 2012;307:1383–93.

18. Huang J, Nair S, Mahoney M, et al. Comparison of FOLFIRI with or without cetuximab in patients with resected stage III colon cancer: NCCTG (Alliance) Intergroup trial N0147. Clin Colorectal Cancer 2014;13:100–9.

19. Efficacy of adjuvant fluorouracil and folinic acid in B2 colon cancer. International Multicentre Pooled Analysis of B2 Colon Cancer Trials (IMPACT B2) Investigators. J Clin Oncol 1999;17:1356–63.

20. Gill S, Loprinzi C, Sargent D, et al. Pooled analysis of fluorouracil-based adjuvant therapy for stage II and III colon cancer: who benefits and by how much? J Clin Oncol 2004;22:1797–806.

21. Gray R, Barnwell J, McConkey C, et al. Adjuvant chemotherapy versus observation in patients with colorectal cancer: a randomised study. Lancet 2007;370:2020–9.

22. Wu X, Zhang J, He X, et al. Postoperative adjuvant chemotherapy for stage II colorectal cancer: a systematic review of 12 randomized controlled trials. J Gastrointestinal Surg 2012;16:646–55.

23. Benson A, Schrag D, Somerfield M, et al. American Society of Clinical Oncology recommendations on adjuvant chemotherapy for stage II colon cancer. J Clin Oncol 2004;22:3408–19.

24. Ribic C, Sargent D, Moore M, et al. Tumor microsatellite-instability status as a predictor of benefit from fluorouracil-based adjuvant chemotherapy for colon cancer. N Engl J Med 2003;349:247–57.

25. Sargent D, Marsoni S, Monges G, et al. Defective mismatch repair as a predictive marker for lack of efficacy of fluorouracil-based adjuvant therapy in colon cancer. J Clin Oncol 2010;28:3219–26.

26. Hutchins G, Southward K, Handley K, et al. Value of mismatch repair, KRAS, and BRAF mutations in predicting recurrence and benefits from chemotherapy in colorectal cancer. J Clin Oncol 2011;29:1261–70.

27. Lai L, Fuller C, Kachnic L, et al. Can pelvic radiotherapy be omitted in select patients with rectal cancer. Seminar Oncol 2006;33:S70–4.

28. Gunderson L, Sargent D, Tepper J, et al. Impact of T and N stage and treatment on survival and relapse in adjuvant rectal cancer: a pooled analysis. J Clin Oncol 2004;22:1785–96.

29. O'Connell J, Martenson J, Wieand H, et al. Improving adjuvant therapy for rectal cancer by combining protracted-infusion fluorouracil with radiation therapy after curative surgery. N Engl J Med 1994;331:502–7.

30. Hofheinz R, Wenz F, Post S, et al. Chemoradiotherapy with capecitabine versus fluorouracil for locally advanced rectal cancer: a randomised, multicentre, non-interiority, phase 3 trial. Lancet Oncol 2012;13:579–88.

31. Tepper J, O'Connell J, Niedzwiecki D, et al. Adjuvant therapy in rectal cancer: analysis of stage, sex, and local control-final report of Intergroup 0114. J Clin Oncol 2002;20:1744–50.

32. Sauer R, Liersch T, Merkel S, et al. Preoperative versus postoperative chemoradiotherapy for locally advanced rectal cancer: results of the German CAO/ARO/AIO-94 randomized phase III trial after a median follow-up of 11 years. J Clin Oncol 2012;30:1926–33.

33. Shandra B, Glas A, Slors F, et al. Rectal cancer: local staging and assessment of lymph node involvement with endoluminal US, CT and MRI imaging–a meta-analysis. Radiology 2004;232:773–83.

34. Wu J. Rectal cancer staging. Clin Colon and Rectal Surg 2007;20:148–57.

35. Guillem J, Diaz-Gonzalez J, Minsky B, et al. cT3N0 rectal cancer: potential overtreatment with preoperative chemotherapy is warranted. J Clin Oncol 2008;26:368–73.

36. Adam I, Mohamdee M, Martin I, et al. Role of circumferential margin involvement in the local recurrence of rectal cancer. Lancet 2006;344:707–11.

37. Park I, You Y, Agarwal A, et al. Neoadjuvant treatment response as an early response indicator for patients with rectal cancer. J Clin Oncol 2012;30:1770–6.

38. Agarwal A, Chang G, Hu CY, Taggart M, Rashid A. Quantified pathologic response assessed as residual tumor burden is a predictor of recurrence-free survival in patients with rectal cancer who undergo resection after neoadjuvant chemoradiotherapy. Cancer 2013;119:4231–41.

39. Aschele C, Cionini L, Lonardi S, et al. Primary tumor response to preoperative chemoradiation with or without oxaliplatin in locally advanced rectal cancer: pathologic results of the STAR-01 randomized phase III trial. J Clin Oncol 2011;29:2773–80.

40. Rodel C, Liersch T, Becker H, et al. Preoperative chemoradiotherapy and post-operative chemotherapy with fluorouracil and oxaliplatin versus fluorouracil along in locally advanced rectal cancer: initial results of the German CAO/ARO/AIO-04 randomised phase III trial. Lancet Oncol 2012;13:679–87.

41. O'Connell J, Colangelo L, Beart R, et al. Capecitabine and oxaliplatin in the preoperative multimodality treatment of rectal cancer: surgical endpoints from

National Surgical Adjuvant Breast and Bowel Project trial R-04. J Clin Oncol 2014;32:1927–34.

42. Gerard J, Azria D, Gourgou-Bourgade S, et al. Clinical outcome of the ACCORD 12/0405 PRODIGE 2 randomized trial in rectal cancer. J Clin Oncol 2012;30:4558–65.

43. Rodel C, Liersch T, Rietkau R, et al. Preoperative chemoradiotherapy and post-operative chemotherapy with 5-fluorouracil and oxaliplatin versus 5-fluorouracil alone in locally advanced rectal cancer: results of the German CAO/ARO/AIO-04 randomized phase III trial. J Clin Oncol 2014;32 [abstract: 3500].

44. Schmoll H, Haustermans K, Price T, et al. Preoperative chemoradiotherapy and postoperative chemotherapy with capecitabine and oxaliplatin versus capecitabine alone in locally advanced rectal cancer: disease-free survival results at interim analysis. J Clin Oncol 2014;32 [abstract:3501].

45. Illum H. Current status of radiosensitizing agents for the management of rectal cancer. Crit Rev Oncog 2012;17:345–59.

46. Smalley S, Benedetti J, Williamson S, et al. Phase III trial of fluorouracil-based chemotherapy regimens plus radiotherapy in postoperative adjuvant rectal cancer: GI INT-0144. J Clin Oncol 2006;24:3542–7.

47. Petersen S, Harling H, Kirkeby L, et al. Postoperative adjuvant chemotherapy in rectal cancer operated for cure. Cochrane Database Syst Rev 2012;(3):CD004078.

48. de Gramont A, Bosset J, Milan C, et al. Randomized trial comparing monthly low-dose leucovorin and fluorouracil bolus with bimonthly high-dose leucovorin and fluorouracil bolus plus continuous infusion for advanced colorectal cancer. A French Intergroup study. J Clin Oncol 1997;15:808–15.

49. Hoff P, Ansari R, Batist G, et al. Comparison of oral capecitabine versus intravenous fluorouracil plus leucovorin as first-line treatment in 605 patients with metastatic colorectal cancer: results of a randomized phase III study. J Clin Oncol 2001;19:2282–92.

50. Van Cutsem E, Hoff P, Harper P, et al. Oral capecitabine vs intravenous 5-fluorouracil and leucovorin: integrated efficacy data and novel analyses from two large, randomised, phase III trials. Br J Cancer 2004;90.

51. Madi A, Fisher D, Wilson R, et al. Oxaliplatin/capecitabine vs oxaliplatin/infusional 5-FU in advanced colorectal cancer: the MRC COIN trial. Br J Cancer 2012;107:1037–43.

52. Seymour M, Thompson L, Wasan H, et al. Chemotherapy options in elderly and frail patients with metastatic colorectal cancer (MRC FOCUS2): an open-label, randomized factorial trial. Lancet 2011;377:1749–59.

53. Cassidy J, Saltz L, Twelves C, et al. Efficacy of capecitabine versus 5-fluorouracil in colorectal and gastric cancers: a meta-analysis of individual data from 6171 patients. Ann Oncol 2011;22:2604–9.

54. Jager E, Heike M, Bernhard O, et al. Weekly high-dose leucovorin versus low-dose leucovorin combined with fluorouracil in advanced colorectal cancer: results of a randomized multicenter trial. J Clin Oncol 1996;14:2274–9.

55. O'Connell M. Phase III trial of 5-fluorouracil and leucovorin in the treatment of advanced colorectal cancer. A Mayo Clinic/North Central Cancer Treatment Group study. Cancer 1989;63:1026–30.

56. Leichman C, Fleming T, Muggia F, et al. Phase II study of fluorouracil and its modulation in advanced colorectal cancer: a Southwest Oncology Group study. J Clin Oncol 1995;13:1303–11.

57. Diaz-Rubio E, Sastre J, Zaniboni A, et al. Oxaliplatin as single agent in previously untreated colorectal carcinoma patients: a phase II multicentric study. Ann Oncol 1998;9:105–8.

58. Becouarn Y, Rougier P. Clinical efficacy of oxaliplatin monotherapy: phase II trials in advanced colorectal cancer. Semin Oncol 1998;25:23–31.
59. Saltz L. Irinotecan in the first-line treatment of colorectal cancer. Oncology 1998; 12:54–8.
60. de Gramont A, Figer A, Seymour M, et al. Leucovorin and fluorouracil with or without oxaliplatin as first-line treatment in advanced colorectal cancer. J Clin Oncol 2000;18:2938–47.
61. Cassidy J, Clarke S, Diaz-Rubio E, et al. XELOX vs FOLFOX-4 as first-line therapy for metastatic colorectal cancer: N016966 updated results. Br J Cancer 2011;105:58–64.
62. Cassidy J, Clarke S, Diaz-Rubio E, et al. Randomized phase III study of capecitabine plus oxaliplatin compared with fluorouracil/folinic acid plus oxaliplatin as first line therapy for metastatic colorectal cancer. J Clin Oncol 2008;26: 2006–12.
63. Goldberg R, Sargent D, Morton R, et al. Randomized controlled trial of reduced-dose bolus fluorouracil plus leucovorin and irinotecan or infused fluorouracil plus leucovorin and oxaliplatin in patients with previously untreated metastatic colorectal cancer: a North American Intergroup trial. J Clin Oncol 2006;24: 3347–53.
64. Pectasides D, Papaxoinis G, Kalogeras K, et al. XELIRI-bevacizumab versus FOLFIRI-bevacizumab as first-line treatment in patients with metastatic colorectal cancer: a Hellenic Cooperative Oncology Group phase III trial with collateral biomarker analysis. BMC Cancer 2012;12:271.
65. Koopman M, Antonini N, Douma J, et al. Sequential versus combination chemotherapy with capecitabine, irinotecan, and oxaliplatin in advanced colorectal cancer (CAIRO): a phase III randomised controlled trial. Lancet 2007;370: 135–42.
66. Kohne C, De Greve J, Hartmann J, et al. Irinotecan combined with infusional 5-fluorouracil/folinic acid or capecitabine plus celecoxib or placebo in the first-line treatment of patients with metastatic colorectal cancer. EORTC study 40015. Ann Oncol 2008;19:920–6.
67. Fuchs C, Marshall J, Mitchell E, et al. Randomized, controlled trial of irinotecan plus infusional, bolus, or oral fluoropyrimidines in first-line treatment of metastatic colorectal cancer: results from the BICC-C study. J Clin Oncol 2007;25: 4779–86.
68. Tournigand C, Andre T, Achille E, et al. FOLFIRI followed by FOLFOX6 or the reverse sequence in advanced colorectal cancer: a randomized GERCOR study. J Clin Oncol 2004;22:229–37.
69. Sargent D, Kohne C, Sanoff H, et al. Pooled safety and efficacy analysis examining the effect of performance status on outcomes in nine first-line treatment trials using individual data from patients with metastatic colorectal cancer. J Clin Oncol 2009;27:1948–55.
70. Ducreux M, Malka D, Mendibourne J, et al. Sequential versus combination chemotherapy for the treatment of advanced colorectal cancer (FFCD 2000-05): an open-label, randomised, phase 3 trial. Lancet Oncol 2011;12:1032–44.
71. Seymour M, Maughan T, Ledermann J, et al. Different strategies of sequential and combination chemotherapy for patients with poor prognosis advanced colorectal cancer (MRC FOCUS): a randomised controlled trial. Lancet 2007; 370:143–52.
72. Grothey A, Sargent D. Overall survival of patients with advanced colorectal cancer correlates with availability of fluorouracil, irinotecan, and oxaliplatin

regardless of whether doublet or single agent therapy is used first line. J Clin Oncol 2005;23:9441–2.

73. Hurwitz H, Fehrenbacher L, Novotny W, et al. Bevacizumab plus irinotecan, fluorouracil, and leucovorin for metastatic colorectal cancer. N Engl J Med 2004; 350:2335–42.

74. Kabbinavar F, Hambleton J, Mass R. Combined analysis of efficacy: the addition of bevacizumab to fluorouracil/leucovorin improves survival in patients with metastatic colorectal cancer. J Clin Oncol 2005;23:3706–12.

75. Hochster H, Hart L, Ramanathan R, et al. Safety and efficacy of oxaliplatin and fluoropyrimidine regimens with or without bevacizumab as first-line treatment for metastatic colorectal cancer: results of the TREE study. J Clin Oncol 2008;21:3523–9.

76. Saltz L, Lenz H, Kindler H, et al. Randomized phase II trial of cetuximab, bevacizumab, and irinotecan compared with cetuximab and bevacizumab alone in irinotecan-refractory colorectal cancer: the BOND-2 study. J Clin Oncol 2007; 25:4557–61.

77. Fuchs C, Marshall J, Barrueco J. Randomized controlled trial of irinotecan plus infusional, bolus, or oral fluoropyrimidines in first-line treatment of metastatic colorectal cancer: updated results from the BICC-C study. J Clin Oncol 2008; 26:689–90.

78. Sobrero A, Ackland S, Clarke S, et al. Phase IV study of bevacizumab in combination with infusional fluorouracil, leucovorin and irinotecan (FOLFIRI) in first-line metastatic colorectal cancer. Oncology 2009;77:113–9.

79. Saltz L, Clarke S, Diaz-Rubio E, et al. Bevacizumab in combination with oxaliplatin-based chemotherapy as first-line therapy in metastatic cancer: a randomized phase III study. J Clin Oncol 2008;26:2013–9.

80. Ranpura V, Hapani S, Wu S, et al. Treatment-related mortality with bevacizumab in cancer patients: a meta-analysis. JAMA 2011;305:487–94.

81. Kohne C, Mineur L, Greil R, et al. First line panitumumab with irinotecan/ 5-fluorouracil/leucovorin treatment in patients with metastatic colorectal cancer. J Cancer Res Clin Oncol 2010;138:65–72.

82. Van Cutsem E, Kohne C, Hitre E, et al. Cetuximab and chemotherapy as initial treatment for metastatic colorectal cancer. N Engl J Med 2009;360:1408–17.

83. Douillard J, Siena S, Cassidy J, et al. Randomized phase III trial of panitumumab with infusional fluorouracil, leucovorin and oxaliplatin (FOLFOX4) versus FOLFOX4 alone as first-line treatment in patients with previously untreated metastatic colorectal cancer: the PRIME study. J Clin Oncol 2010;28:4697–705.

84. Petrelli N, Borgonovo K, Barni S. The predictive role of skin rash with cetuximab and panitumumab in colorectal cancer patients: a systemic review and meta-analysis. Target Oncol 2013;8:173–81.

85. Dahabreh I, Terasawa T, Castaldi P, et al. Anti-epidermal growth factor receptor treatment effect modification by KRAS mutations in advanced colorectal cancer. Ann Intern Med 2011;154:37–9.

86. Douillard J, Oliner K, Siena S, et al. Panitumumab-FOLFOX4 treatment and RAS mutations in colorectal cancer. N Engl J Med 2013;369:1023–34.

87. Tze-Kiong E, Chen C, Bujanda L, et al. Current approaches for predicting a lack of response to anti-EGFR therapy in KRAS wild-type patients. Biomed Res Int 2014;2014:591867.

88. Tveit K, Guren T, Glimelius B, et al. Phase III trial of cetuximab with continuous or intermittent fluorouracil, leucovorin, and oxaliplatin (Nordic FLOX) versus FLOX alone in first-line treatment of metastatic colorectal cancer: the NORDIC-VII study. J Clin Oncol 2012;15:1755–62.

89. Maughan T, Adams R, Smith C, et al. Addition of cetuximab to oxaliplatin-based first-line combination chemotherapy for treatment of advanced colorectal cancer: results of the randomised phase 3 MRC COIN trial. Lancet 2011;377:2103–14.

90. Bokemeyer C, Bondarenko I, Hartmann JT, et al. Efficacy according to biomarker status of cetuximab plus FOLFOX4 as first-line treatment of metastatic colorectal cancer: the OPUS study. Ann Oncol 2011;22(7):1535–46.

91. Heinemann V, von Weikersthal LF, Decker T, et al. FOLFIRI plus cetuximab versus FOLFIRI plus bevacizumab as first-line treatment for patients with metastatic colorectal cancer (FIRE-3): a randomised, open-label, phase 3 trial. Lancet Oncol 2014;15(10):1065–75.

92. Falcone A, Ricci S, Brunetti I, et al. Phase III trial of infusional fluorouracil, leucovorin, oxaliplatin, and irinotecan (FOLFOXIRI) compared with infusional fluorouracil, leucovorin, and irinotecan (FOLFIRI) as first-line treatment for metastatic colorectal cancer: the Gruppo Oncologico Nord. J Clin Oncol 2007;25:1670–6.

93. Souglakos J, Androulakis N, Syrigos K, et al. FOLOXIRI (folinic acid, 5-fluorouracil, oxaliplatin and irinotecan) vs FOLFIRI (folinic acid, 5-fluorouracil and irinotecan) as first line treatment in metastatic colorectal cancer (MCC): a multicentre randomised phase III trial from the Hellenic Oncology Research Group (HORG). Br J Cancer 2006;94:798–805.

94. Falcone A, Cremolini C, Masi G, et al. FOLFOXIRI/bevacizumab versus FOLFIRI/BEV as first-line treatment in unresectable metastatic colorectal cancer (mCRC) patients (pts): results of the phase III TRIBE trial by GONO group. J Clin Oncol 2013;31 [abstract: 3505].

95. Van Cutsem E, Kohne C, Lang I, et al. Cetuximab plus irinotecan, fluorouracil and leucovorin as first line treatment for metastatic colorectal cancer: updated analysis of overall survival according to tumor KRAS and BRAF mutation status. J Clin Oncol 2011;29:2011–9.

96. Gruenberger T, Bridgewater J, Chau I, et al. Randomized phase II study of bevacizumab with mFOLFOX6 or FOLFOXIRI in patients with initially unresectable liver metastases from colorectal cancer: resectability and safety in OLIVIA. J Clin Oncol 2013;31 [abstract: 3619].

97. Folprecht G, Hamann S, Schutte K, et al. Dose escalating study of cetuximab and 5-FU/folinic acid/oxaliplatin/iriniotecan (FOLFOXIRI) in first line therapy of patients with metastatic colorectal cancer. BMC Cancer 2014;14:521.

98. Fornaro L, Lonardi S, Masi G, et al. FOLFOXIRI in combination with panitumumab as first-line treatment in quadruple wild-type (KRAS, NRAS, HRAS, BRAF) metastatic colorectal cancer patients: a phase II trial by the Gruppo Oncologico Nord Ovest (GONO). Ann Oncol 2013;24:2062–7.

99. Saltz L, Badarinath S, Dakhil S, et al. Phase III trial of cetuximab, bevacizumab, and 5-fluorouracil/leucovorin vs FOLFOX-bevacizumab in colorectal cancer. Clin Colorectal Cancer 2012;11:101–11.

100. Tol J, Koopman M, Cats A, et al. Chemotherapy, bevacizumab, and cetuximab in metastatic colorectal cancer. N Engl J Med 2009;360:563–72.

101. Hecht R, Mitchell E, Chidiac T, et al. A randomized phase IIIB trial of chemotherapy, bevacizumab, and panitumumab compared with chemotherapy and bevacizumab alone for metastatic colorectal cancer. J Clin Oncol 2009;27:672–80.

102. Larsen F, Pfeiffer P, Nielsen D, et al. Bevacizumab in combination with cetuximab and irinotecan after failure of cetuximab and irinotecan in patients with metastatic colorectal cancer. Acta Oncol 2011;50:574–7.

103. Batlle F, Cuadrado E, Castro J, et al. Irinotecan-cetuximab-bevacizumab as salvage treatment in heavily pretreated metastatic colorectal cancer patients: a retrospective observational study. Chemotherapy 2011;57:138–44.

104. Kweekel D, Guchelaar H, Gelderblom H. Clinical and pharmacogenetic factors associated with irinotecan toxicity. Cancer Treat Rev 2008;34:656–69.

105. Colucci G, Gebbia V, Paoletti G, et al. Phase III randomized trial of FOLFIRI versus FOLFOX in the treatment of advanced colorectal cancer: a multicenter study of the Gruppo Oncologico Dell'Italia Meridionale. J Clin Oncol 2005;23: 4866–75.

106. Engstrom P, National Comprehensive Cancer Network. Systemic therapy for advanced or metastatic colorectal cancer; National Comprehensive Cancer Network guidelines for combining anti-vascular endothelial growth factor and anti-epidermal growth factor receptor monoclonal antibodies with chemotherapy. Pharmacotherapy 2008;28:18S–22S.

107. Heinemann V, von Weikersthal L, Decker T, et al. Randomized comparison of FOLFIRI plus cetuximab versus FOLFIRI plus bevacizumab as first-line treatment of KRAS wild type metastatic colorectal cancer: German AIO study KRK-0306. J Clin Oncol 2013;31(Suppl) [abstract: LBA3506].

108. Adam R, Delvart V, Pascal G, et al. Rescue surgery for unresectable colorectal liver metastases downstaged by chemotherapy: a model to predict long-term survival. Ann Surg 2004;240:644–57.

109. Vauthey J, Pawlik T, Ribero D, et al. Chemotherapy regimen predicts steatohepatitis and an increase in 90 day mortality after surgery for hepatic colorectal metastases. J Clin Oncol 2006;24:2065–72.

110. Folprecht G, Gruenberger T, Bechstein W, et al. Tumour response and secondary resectability of colorectal liver metastases following neoadjuvant chemotherapy with cetuximab: the CELIM randomized phase 2 trial. Lancet Oncol 2010;11:38–47.

111. Ye L, Liu T, Ren L, et al. Randomized controlled trial of cetuximab plus chemotherapy for patients with KRAS wild-type unresectable colorectal liver-limited metastases. J Clin Oncol 2013;31:1931–8.

112. Petrettli F, Barni S. Resectability and outcome with anti-EGFR agents in patients with KRAS wild-type colorectal liver-limited metastases: a meta-analysis. Int J Colorectal Dis 2012;27:997–1004.

113. Ciliberto D, Prati U, Roveda L, et al. Role of systemic chemotherapy in the management of resected or resectable colorectal liver metastases: a systematic review and meta-analysis of randomized controlled trials. Oncol Rep 2012;27: 1849–56.

114. Benson A, Venook A, Bekaii-Saab T, et al. Colon cancer, version 3.2014. J Natl Compr Canc Netw 2014;12:1028–59.

115. Simkens L, Koopman M, Punt C. Optimal duration of systemic treatment in metastatic colorectal cancer. Curr Opin Oncol 2014;26:448–53.

116. Chibaudel B, Maindrault-Goebel F, Lledo G, et al. Can chemotherapy be discontinued in unresectable metastatic colorectal cancer? The GERCOR OPTIMOX2 study. J Clin Oncol 2009;27:5727–33.

117. Arnold D, Graeven U, Lerchenmuller C, et al. Maintenance strategy with fluoropyrimidines plus bevacizumab, BEV alone, or no treatment as first line treatment for patients with metastatic colorectal cancer: a phase III non-inferiority trial (AIO KRK 0207). J Clin Oncol 2014;32 [abstract: 3503].

118. Koopman M, Simkens L, May A, et al. Maintenance treatment with capecitabine plus bevacizumab versus observation after induction treatment with

chemotherapy + bevacizumab in metastatic colorectal cancer. J Clin Oncol 2014;32(Suppl) [abstract: LBA388].

119. Koeberle D, Betticher D, Von Moos R, et al. Bevacizumab continuation versus no continuation after first-line chemo-bevacizumab therapy in patients with metastatic colorectal cancer: a randomized phase III non-inferiority trial (SAKK 41/06). J Clin Oncol 2013;31(Suppl) [abstract: 3503].

120. Arnold D, Stein A. New developments in the second line treatment of metastatic colorectal cancer: potential place in therapy. Drugs 2013;73:883–91.

121. Bekaii-Saab T, Wu C. Seeing the forest through the trees: a systematic review of the safety and efficacy of combination therapies used in the treatment of metastatic colorectal cancer. Crit Rev Oncol Hematol 2014;91:9–34.

122. Bennouna J, Sastre J, Arnold D, et al. Continuation of bevacizumab after first progression in metastatic colorectal cancer (ML18147): a randomised phase 3 trial. Lancet Oncol 2013;14:29–37.

123. Grothey A, Van Cutsem E, Sobrero A, et al. Regorafenib monotherapy for previously treated metastatic colorectal cancer (CORRECT): an international, multicentre, randomised, placebo-controlled, phase 3 trial. Lancet 2013;381:303–12.

124. Van Cutsem E, Tabernero J, Lakomy R, et al. The addition of aflibercept to fluorouracil, leucovorin and irinotecan improves survival in a phase III randomized trial in patients with metastatic colorectal cancer previously treated with an oxaliplatin-based regimen. J Clin Oncol 2014;30:3499–506.

125. Porschen R, Arkenau H, Kubicka S, et al. Phase III study of capecitabine plus oxaliplatin compared with fluorouracil and leucovorin plus oxaliplatin in metastatic colorectal cancer: a final report of the AIO Colorectal Study Group. J Clin Oncol 2007;25:4217–23.

126. Ashley A, Sargent D, Alberts S, et al. Updated efficacy and toxicity analysis of irinotecan and oxaliplatin (IROX). Cancer 2007;199:670–7.

Ablative and Catheter-Directed Therapies for Colorectal Liver and Lung Metastases

 CrossMark

Elena N. Petre, MD*, Constantinos T. Sofocleous, MD, PhD, Stephen B. Solomon, MD

KEYWORDS

- Interventional radiology • Colorectal liver metastases • Colorectal lung metastases
- Ablation therapy • Intra-arterial therapy

KEY POINTS

- Interventional radiologists play an important role in the multidisciplinary care of patients with colorectal cancer with liver metastases.
- Ablation therapy can focally destroy liver metastases, providing long-term survival in select cases.
- The "test-of-time" approach with ablation before hepatic metastatectomy can help select patients who will benefit from surgery and patients whose biology will lead to innumerable metastases, making them ultimately not a good surgical candidate.
- Intra-arterial therapies with chemoembolization, radioembolization, drug-eluting beads, and intra-arterial chemotherapy can play a role in patients with unresectable liver metastases and liver-dominant disease.

INTRODUCTION

Treatment of limited metastatic disease can prolong survival; however, in many instances patients may not be ideally suited for surgery, may not be able to discontinue chemotherapy in the perioperative period, or may prefer a less invasive therapy to maintain quality of life. Several image-guided procedures have evolved within the last 10 years that allow the management of limited metastatic disease in nonresectable patients and those that have recurred after resection. These locoregional therapies include local tumor ablation and catheter-directed therapies, and can occasionally downstage a patient with inoperable metastases to an operable status. Ablative therapies cause focal destruction of tissue, and have increasingly been shown to

Department of Radiology, Interventional Radiology Service, Memorial Sloan Kettering Cancer Center, 1275 York Avenue, H-118, New York, NY 10065, USA
* Corresponding author.
E-mail address: petree@mskcc.org

Hematol Oncol Clin N Am 29 (2015) 117–133
http://dx.doi.org/10.1016/j.hoc.2014.09.007
0889-8588/15/$ – see front matter © 2015 Elsevier Inc. All rights reserved.

successfully eradicate colorectal liver metastases. Although it has been less used than hepatic ablation, pulmonary thermal ablation has achieved promising results with respect to safety and local tumor control. An increasing number of studies evaluating local ablation for the treatment of pulmonary colorectal metastases is emerging. Definitive integration of ablative therapies into the management of metastatic colorectal cancer depends on defining the patient population in which ablation can be used instead of surgery with equivalent results. In hepatocellular carcinoma, for example, the data have suggested that for tumors smaller than 2 cm ablation may be preferable to surgery.[1] With improving technology, similar equivalencies with ablation in colorectal metastases may arise. Catheter-directed therapies such as transarterial chemoembolization (TACE), drug-eluting beads (DEB), selective internal radiation therapy (SIRT), and intra-arterial chemotherapy ports are all potential techniques for managing the patient with unresectable liver metastases.

ABLATIVE THERAPY FOR COLORECTAL LIVER METASTASES

Hepatectomy with curative intent is the treatment of choice for colorectal liver metastases (CLM), although only 20% of patients are resectable at presentation.[2] Five-year survival rates after complete resection of CLM range from 35% to 58%.[3,4] For unresectable patients, median survival ranges from 6 months without any treatment to 12 to 24 months for patients receiving first-line and second-line chemotherapy.[5–7] Ablation technologies cause focal destruction of tissue. Several ablative tools are currently used for the treatment of colorectal cancer metastases, including radiofrequency ablation (RFA), microwave ablation (MWA), cryoablation, laser ablation, and focused ultrasound ablation, all of which rely on extreme heat or cold to produce cell death and exact tissue damage.[8] A nonthermal ablation technique, irreversible electroporation (IRE), uses electrical fields to cause cell death without apparently harming tissue protein architecture that makes up structures such as bile ducts and vessels. This newer technique may open up new ablative opportunities near critical structures that would otherwise not be possible to ablate safely with thermal energy.

The advantages of ablation techniques derive from their being less invasive and, consequently, less morbid than surgical resection. Patients can generally be treated as outpatients, with a rapid recovery to normal activities. Ablative therapies minimize the destruction of healthy liver tissue in comparison with hepatic resection. This parameter is an important one for patients with underlying cirrhosis or steatohepatitis from prolonged chemotherapy exposure, and those who have previously undergone extensive liver resection. Percutaneous ablation procedures can be repeated to treat recurrences as needed, with minimal loss of unaffected parenchyma. As such, ablation can be used to salvage some recurrences after resection.[9,10] Whereas chemotherapy routines are frequently interrupted for 6 weeks by surgical resection, this same requirement is not present with percutaneous ablation techniques.[11]

RFA is the most widely used and well-studied ablation modality. RFA has been used to control CLM successfully in selected patients with nonresectable disease.[12–16] There is an overall recognition that for small tumors that can be ablated completely with clear margins, RFA may be able to provide results similar to those of surgery,[17–19] despite the fact that ablation series included patients with major medical comorbidities, insufficient hepatic reserve for surgery, extrahepatic disease, or tumors located in proximity to major vascular structures.[20–25] In addition, the long survival times after curative surgery may reflect selection bias of early detection of CLM. These results support the use of thermal ablation as a procedure with curative intent, similarly to surgical metastasectomy, for selected patients with small size and number of CLM that can be ablated with appropriate margins. To date, a randomized study for resectable liver metastases comparing resection with RFA has not been completed.[26]

A key component of a successful ablation is the creation of an effective ablation zone that will encompass the target lesion with clear margins (ideally 1 cm all around the target tumor). Imaging guidance during the procedure is critical to ensure adequate targeting and evaluate for completeness of the ablation (**Fig. 1**). The ablation zone should not enhance, and should be larger than the target tumor accounting for the desired margin.

Median overall survival (OS) times beyond 30 months after thermal ablation are superior when compared with unresectable historical controls treated by chemotherapy,[13,27,28] but these findings can be biased by patient selection. However, it is not uncommon that patients undergo thermal ablation only after they have failed several lines of chemotherapy. Prospective randomized trials are essential in this case as well, to evaluate the exact benefit of tumor ablation therapies over systemic chemotherapy. As yet there is a single randomized clinical trial comparing RFA combined with systemic chemotherapy with systemic chemotherapy alone as first-line therapy for CLM.[29] The benefit of RFA in combination with systemic chemotherapy is reflected in a statistically significant prolongation of median progression-free survival (PFS) to 16.8 months for the combined arm, compared with 9.9 months for the chemotherapy-only arm. Overall patient survival was 61.7% for the combined therapy and 57.6% for the chemotherapy-only control group at 30 months. This modest

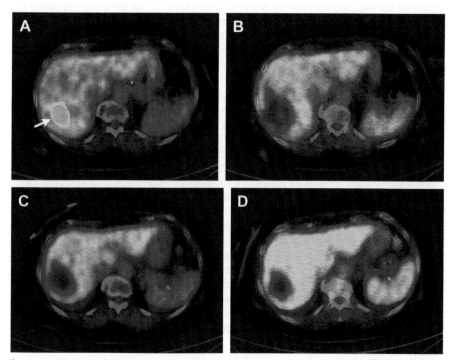

Fig. 1. An 82-year-old woman with metastatic colorectal cancer. (*A*) Fused ^{18}F-fluorodeoxyglucose (FDG) PET/CT before ablation procedure shows liver metastasis in segment 5/6 (*arrow*); this was treated with radiofrequency ablation (RFA) (not shown) (*B*) Fused FDG-PET/CT at the end of the ablation procedure shows the ablation zone with no metabolic activity. (*C*) Fused PET/CT images show a good ablation result at 3 months after RFA. (*D*) There is a further decrease in the size of the ablation zone and no metabolic activity at 6 months.

prolongation did not reach significance in a study that was not powered to address this and with a follow-up time of only 30 months.

Results from long-term follow-up (up to 10 years) are now available from a retrospective study.[19] These results (5-, 7-, and 10-year OS rates of 47.8%, 25%, and 18%, respectively) are essentially equivalent to those of surgical resection. Survival was significantly improved in patients who underwent repeat ablation after local tumor progression (45.5 months vs 31 months for patients who were not retreated).[19]

The local recurrence rate after RFA varies widely between 2%[30] and 60%,[31] and remains an important limitation of RFA,[30–35] especially when compared with resection. Size of the lesion, location from major vessels, and ablation margin are key factors that have been associated with local tumor control. A tumor size greater than 3 cm is now known to be associated with a higher rate of local progression after RFA.[36–38] Tumors adjacent to vessels larger than 3 mm have an increased risk of local recurrence, because thermal energy is dissipated away from the target tumor as a result of adjacent blood flow (the so-called heat-sink phenomenon).[36,38–40] Like the surgical margin,[41] the size of the ablation margin has been associated with local tumor control.[36,42–44]

Cryotherapy alone or in combination with hepatic resection has been used in selected patients, with oncologic outcomes comparable with surgery.[45,46] Cryoablation applied to the edge of hepatic resections (edge cryotherapy) is frequently used in cases with "close" margins, affording a 5-year survival rate of 31% for advanced colorectal cancer, as reported by Ng and colleagues.[47] The same investigators reported a 5-year survival rate of 21% for the group treated with hepatic cryotherapy alone or in combination with liver resection, with curative intention.[47] These results are promising, and suggest that this method can afford a potential cure for selected cases of advanced CLM not amenable to curative surgery with hepatectomy alone.

Test of Time

In selected resectable patients, percutaneous ablation was proposed with the concept of the "test of time."[35] Using this approach, selected resectable patients with small-volume disease that can be ablated with margins underwent percutaneous ablation while being observed and imaged, with the intention to undergo hepatic metastasectomy. This delayed period allows the biology of disease to express itself. Patients completely treated by ablation without local recurrence, in addition to those who develop multifocal unresectable metastases, are spared unnecessary surgery. For patients with local recurrence or limited intrahepatic progression, there would still be an opportunity to repeat ablation or undergo metastasectomy. The test-of-time approach could represent the starting point in prospective randomized trials comparing percutaneous ablation with surgery that will support the use of ablation as the first-line treatment of CLM in selected cases. One other practical application of the test-of-time approach is for the treatment of recurrent CLM after hepatic resection (particularly new liver metastasis within 6 months of resection) in patients who are technically re-resectable. Patients with successful ablation and those who would have further recurrences benefit from avoiding the increased morbidity of nonbeneficial re-resection.

Newer Technologies: Microwave Ablation and Irreversible Electroporation

MWA was developed to overcome some of the limitations of RFA. MWA may provide larger and more uniform ablation volumes in a shorter time and higher rates of complete ablation, owing to avoidance of the heat-sink effect. MWA has demonstrated its superiority over RFA in treating larger tumors, resulting in lower recurrence rates (as low as 6%).[48] With regard to OS, intraoperative MWA has produced results similar to those of surgery in retrospective series, up to a median of 43 months.[49,50] To date there is a single randomized trial comparing microwave ablation with hepatic resection in patients with CLM.[51] The mean survival time was 27 months in the MWA group, compared with 25 months in the surgery group. The mean disease-free interval was 11.3 months in the MWA group versus 13.3 months in the surgery group. These differences were not statistically significant. This trial was underpowered to determine differences in survival between the groups, owing to the small sample size (40 patients, from which 10 were excluded after randomization).

IRE is generally indicated for tumors that are deemed inappropriate for thermal ablation because of the relatively high risk of collateral damage caused by tumor proximity to bile ducts or other structures that would be injured by the heat. Clinical series that included patients with CLM have demonstrated a primary efficacy of 67% to 100% for tumors adjacent to major vascular/biliary structures.[52–55] The risk of recurrence seems to be higher for tumors greater than 3 cm in size.[52–54] Current evidence, while encouraging, is still limited, with no randomized controlled trials. Most of the series included different organs and differing pathology, making it difficult to draw any generalized conclusions.

CATHETER-DIRECTED LIVER THERAPIES

Arterial therapies for colorectal liver cancer metastases can be performed to complement or salvage the effects of systemic therapy. The concept of intra-arterial therapies relies on the fact that liver cancers derive their blood supply predominantly from hepatic arteries, whereas normal liver parenchyma has a predominantly portal vein source of blood supply.[56] The most common techniques of intra-arterial therapies for CLM include intra-arterial hepatic chemotherapy (IAHC), TACE, and SIRT with yttrium-90–impregnated microspheres. Two more therapies are available, namely intraportal drug delivery and isolated liver perfusion.

Intra-arterial Hepatic Chemotherapy

IAHC aims to increase the drug concentration in liver metastases and thereby improve response rates.[57] This approach can be best applied with drugs having a high first-pass effect. One drug that has been extensively used is floxuridine (FUDR), which has a first-pass extraction rate of 95% and can increase the liver dose by 100 to 300 times higher than the systemic perfusion.[58,59] Historically, repeated or continuous IAHC has been delivered by a catheter and pump system requiring laparotomy. More recently, IAHC has become deliverable via an interventional radiology approach with a subcutaneous port placed.[60] In one study of 36 patients with extensive nonresectable liver metastases (ie, ≥ 4 metastases in 86% and bilobar in 91%) using IAHC with oxaliplatin (100 mg/m^2 in 2 hours) plus intravenous 5-fluorouracil (5-FU)/leucovorin (LV) (400 mg/m^2 in 2 hours; 5-FU 400 mg/m^2 bolus then 2500 mg/m^2 in 46 hours) and cetuximab (400 mg/m^2 then 250 mg/m^2/wk or 500 mg/m^2 every 2 weeks) as first-line treatment overall response rate was 90% and disease control rate was 100%. Forty-eight percent of patients were downstaged enough to undergo an R0 resection and/or RFA.[56]

Conventional Transarterial Chemoembolization and Transarterial Chemoembolization with Drug-Eluting Beads

There are several different techniques under the acronym TACE. The most common procedure is the intra-arterial injection of chemotherapy emulsified with Lipiodol

Ultra-Fluid (LUF; Laboratoire Guerbet, Aulnay, France) followed by injection of embolic material.[61–65] With Lipiodol-TACE, the ratio of drug concentration in the tumor compared with the healthy liver and peripheral blood levels can be as high as 10 and 1000 times, respectively.[64] Embolization after chemo-Lipiodol increases the efficacy of treatment by prolonging contact of chemotherapy to the tumor cells and by adding ischemia to the highly hypervascularized tumor usually targeted with this treatment. Such embolization has been reported to induce failure of the transmembrane pump, thus increasing drug retention inside the cells.[65]

One group using the regimen of cisplatin, doxorubicin, mitomycin C, ethiodol, and polyvinyl alcohol has shown an overall response rate of 43%.[66] Median survivals of 33 months from initial diagnosis, 27 months from the time of liver metastases, and 9 months from the start of chemoembolization were documented, suggesting a possible improvement over reported survival time for systemic therapies alone.[66] Another group using mitomycin C alone (52.5%), mitomycin C with gemcitabine (33%), or mitomycin C and irinotecan (14.5%) has shown an overall response rate of 63%.[67]

Recently, drug-eluting beads have been developed that allow drug release after the bead has been embolized into the tumor microcirculation. One of the drugs that has been loaded on these beads is irinotecan. The advantage of the beads is a reduced systemic delivery of chemotherapy. Irinotecan-loaded beads had a 75% reduced systemic plasma level compared with intra-arterial irinotecan alone.[68]

In a randomized study of 2 courses of DEBIRI (Biocompatibles, Oxford, CT, USA) (36 patients) compared with 8 courses of intravenous irinotecan, 5-FU, and leucovorin (FOLFIRI; 38 patients) used to treat 74 patients who failed at least 2 lines of chemotherapy, the DEBIRI arm was met with statistically significant improvement of all oncologic outcomes including patient survival.[69] Specifically, the response rates were 69% for the DEBIRI group compared with 30% for the systemic FOLFIRI group. Similarly, the 2-year OS was 56% compared with 32%, and the median OS was 22 months compared with 15 months for DEBIRI versus FOLFIRI groups. Improvement in quality of life was of longer duration for the DEBIRI group (8 months) than for the FOLFIRI group (3 months, $P = .0002$). Finally, overall cost was lower for the DEBIRI treatment arm.

In a multicenter, single-arm study of 55 patients who underwent DEBIRI after failing systemic chemotherapy, response rates were 66% at 6 months and 75% at 12 months, with an OS of 19 months and a PFS of 11 months.[70]

A recent comparison study of DEBIRI versus radioembolization for salvage therapy for liver-dominant CLM including a series of 36 patients reported similar survival for both treatments, with median survival times of 7.7 months for the DEBIRI group and 6.9 months for the radioembolization (SIRT) group. The 1-, 2-, and 5-year survival rates were 43%, 10%, and 0% in the DEBIRI group and 34%, 18%, and 0% in the SIRT group.[71]

Approximately 20% of DEBIRI sessions are associated with adverse events (most commonly CTCAE [Common Terminology Criteria for Adverse Events] grades 1 and 2) during or after the treatment. The factors predictive of adverse events and significantly longer stay in hospital are: lack of pretreatment with hepatic arterial lidocaine ($P = .005$); greater than 3 treatments ($P = .05$); achievement of complete stasis ($P = .04$); treatment with greater than 100 mg DEBIRI in 1 session ($P = .03$); bilirubin greater than 2.0 μg/dL with greater than 50% liver replaced by tumor ($P = .05$).[72]

Radioembolization/Selective Internal Radiation Therapy

Traditional external beam radiation therapy in patients with diffuse hepatic malignancy does not improve OS[73] because liver tolerance for developing radiation-induced injury is low compared with the doses required for tumoricidal effect.[74] The usual dose to treat a tumor is 70 Gy, whereas normal liver tissue tolerance to radiation is 30 Gy.[75] These facts resulted in the idea of selective internal transarterial radiotherapy with the delivery of yttrium-90–impregnated microspheres. Selective intra-arterial delivery enables doses higher than 120 Gy to target the tumor without reaching the liver toxicity threshold. Radioembolization allows delivery of high doses of ionizing radiation to the tumor with minimal radiation to surrounding tissue, thus causing considerably less toxicity to the normal liver.[76] Patients referred to radioembolization have unresectable (and noneligible for ablation) CLM, liver-only or liver-dominant disease, life expectancy of at least 3 months, and acceptable liver reserve. SIRT has been safely used as a salvage therapy in heavily pretreated patients who progressed after multiple lines of systemic and hepatic arterial chemotherapy in addition to resection.[77] Overall response of 17% to 35% and stable disease rates of 24% to 61% have been described.[78,79] Median survival after radioembolization has ranged from 6.7 to 17 months.[80] Modest effects of radioembolization were seen when it was used as a salvage monotherapy after complete failure of chemotherapy. Radioembolization alone in this setting showed an overall response of 24%, a PFS of 3.7 months, and 1- and 2-year overall survival rates of 50.4% and 19.6%, respectively.[81] The major contribution of radioembolization was documented when it was used together with systemic chemotherapy (**Fig. 2**).[82,83] The major concept behind this combined treatment was that tumors were sensitized by one treatment for the other and, thus, a synergistic effect of SIRT with chemotherapy was seen, with better response rates.[84] In a randomized controlled trial the combination of SIRT with protracted 5-FU had a significantly better PFS when compared with protracted 5-FU alone in patients who had previously failed regimens containing 5-FU.[83]

ABLATIVE THERAPY FOR COLORECTAL LUNG METASTASES

Metastasectomy may afford a prolonged survival of up to 60% at 5 years for patients with limited pulmonary metastases from colorectal cancer.[85–88] However, many patients are poor surgical candidates because of compromised pulmonary function, concurrent medical conditions, or previous lung resections. Patients with limited pulmonary metastases will require multiple repeated resections because not all of the metastatic disease is detectable at first presentation and because there is a high likelihood of tumor recurrences. However, repeat thoracotomy is technically challenging and further removes functional pulmonary tissue. In patients with unresectable isolated colorectal lung metastases, a median survival time of 19 months was observed after chemotherapy.[89]

Ablation of pulmonary colorectal metastases is an appealing technique, as it: (1) has a limited effect on pulmonary function; (2) is repeatable; (3) does not interfere with chemotherapy; and (4) maintains patients' quality of life. Several series have shown that RFA can be a safe and effective treatment for unresectable CLM. However, special considerations apply to thermal ablation in lung tissue because of the low thermal and electrical conductivity of air surrounding the tumors, resulting in difficulty in ablating the marginal parenchyma. Similarly to liver ablation, the presence of vessels and airways may result in a heat-sink effect, thus increasing the risk of local recurrence. An ablative margin of at least 5 mm around the tumor should always be the end point of pulmonary RFA (**Fig. 3**). To achieve this, repositioning the electrode multiple times in an overlapping manner is frequently needed, especially for larger tumors.

The local tumor progression rate after lung RFA varies in the literature between 9%[90] and 38%.[91] The size of the ablated tumor was shown to be an independent factor for

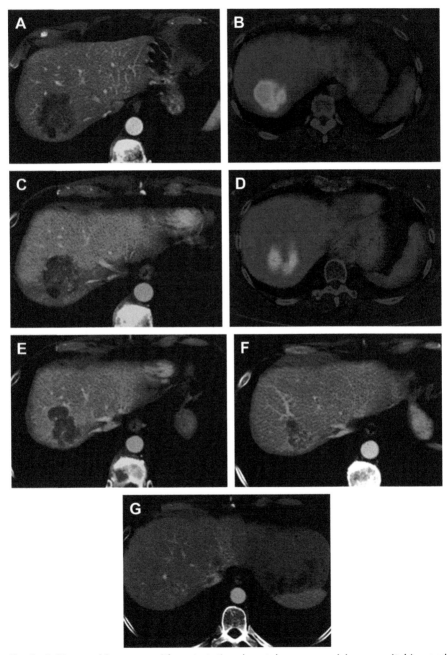

Fig. 2. A 61-year-old woman with metastatic colorectal cancer receiving capecitabine and bevacizumab chemotherapy presented with an increase in size (*A*) and FDG uptake (*B*) of the dominant metastasis in the right hepatic dome. The patient underwent radioembolization, with good response at 3 months as documented by CT (*C*) and PET/CT (*D*). The lesion in the right hepatic dome continued to decrease in size after 6 months (*E*), 12 months (*F*), and 24 months (*G*).

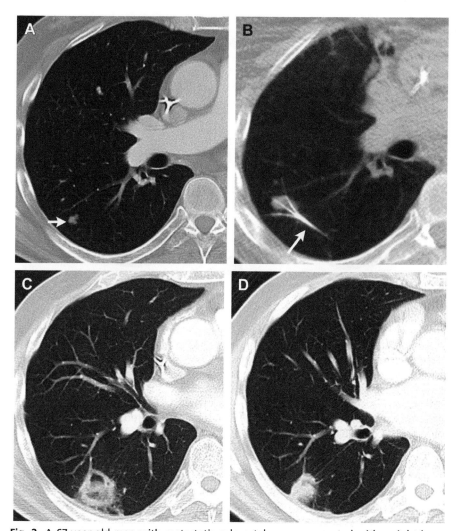

Fig. 3. A 67-year-old man with metastatic colorectal cancer presented with a right lower lobe metastasis (*arrow*) (*A*). (*B*) The patient underwent RFA (*arrow* indicates the ablation needle; image was acquired with the patient in prone position and rotated for comparison purposes). (*C*) Contrast-enhanced CT 4 weeks after RFA shows patchy consolidation, small lucencies, and ground-glass opacity at the ablation site, consistent with postprocedural changes. Follow-up imaging shows continuous decrease in size of the ablation zone after 4 months (*D*) and 9 months (*E*). (*F*) Follow-up CT 14 months after RFA shows a linear opacity with no signs of local tumor progression.

local tumor progression,[91,92] with significantly lower PFS rates for patients in whom the ablated lung metastasis was greater than 3 cm (61% at 1 year and 34% at 3 years vs 88% and 69%, respectively, for tumor size ≤3 cm[92]). A carcinoembryonic antigen level of greater than 5 ng/mL was also associated with decreased local tumor PFS.[91] Median OS of CLM after RFA has been consistently reported to be between 31 and 46 months, with 1-, 2-, and 3-year survival rates of 84% to 95%, 54% to 72%, and 35% to 57%, respectively.[90–95] A lung colorectal metastasis greater than 3 cm was

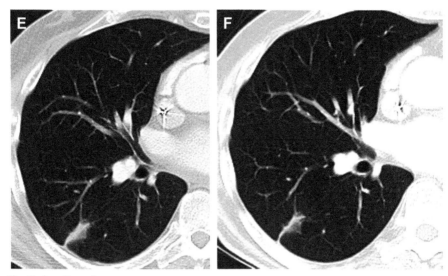

Fig. 3. (*continued*).

independently associated with decreased OS after RFA.[91,92] Patients who undergo ablation of more than 1 growing pulmonary nodule in the setting of other stable lung metastases seem to have a significantly lower OS rate at 3 years after RFA compared with patients treated with RFA to cure 1 (or more) lesion that represents the only pulmonary disease at that time (27% vs 78%, $P = .05$).[94]

Because RFA often has technical challenges resulting from poor electrical conduction in the lung, both cryoablation and MWA are being explored. To date there is only one report of cryoablation for the treatment of pulmonary colorectal metastases.[96] This study included 24 patients with 55 metastatic lung tumors, and reported a median OS of 43 months and a 3-year survival rate of 60%. These findings are very similar to those of RFA. Recently, the safety and efficacy of lung MWA have been prospectively evaluated in nonsurgical candidates with pulmonary metastases.[97] The study included 80 patients with various lung metastases, half of which were of colorectal cancer origin. One- and 2-year survival rates were 91.3% and 75%, respectively, with no significant difference by histopathologic type. Higher survival rates were observed in patients who were tumor-free after ablation than in patients who progressed. Local tumor control rate at 18 months was 73% for the entire group and 76% in the colorectal pulmonary metastases group.[97]

As patients with metastatic colorectal cancer are living longer, the possibility of incorporating chemotherapy breaks into their care without negatively affecting survival has to be considered. Pulmonary ablation of a solitary nodule in the setting of no extrapulmonary disease can afford patients a "chemotherapy holiday" while under rigorous imaging surveillance. Such chemotherapy breaks of up to 20 months were reported to be possible without disease progression.[94]

SUMMARY

Interventional radiologists are playing an increasing role in the management of patients with metastatic colorectal cancer. Implementation of the interventional radiology clinic for consultation has expanded the role of the interventional radiologist as a consultant and as an important contributor to the multidisciplinary management and customization of the treatment of these patients.

In the interventional radiologist's armamentarium are ablative tools that can focally destroy small numbers of liver metastases. Many of the techniques offer minimally invasive treatments that maintain quality of life, do not interfere with chemotherapy regimens, and are repeatable as needed.

In view of the established impact of surgical morbidity on survival[98,99] and the improved safety profile of ablation, selected patients with lesions that could be ablated with sufficient margins may benefit from the least invasive and equally effective ablative therapy. The use of ablation in a test-of-time paradigm may limit unnecessary and morbid resections, significantly contributing to the preservation of patients' quality of life.

Locoregional arterially directed therapies for liver-dominant metastases allow the interventional radiology physician to manage the unresectable patient with the aim of extending disease-free periods and OS and, hopefully, converting him or her to a resection candidate for a potential cure. In particular, IAHC and SIRT have reported a fraction of treated patients being downstaged to resection. Both IAHC and SIRT have also been associated with best oncologic outcomes when combined with earlier lines of systemic chemotherapy.[100]

As all of these tools and techniques have become available and have been perfected over the past decade, it will become important for them to be investigated in clinical trials to best determine their appropriate use in the care of the colorectal patient with liver or lung metastases. The selection of the best therapy for each patient requires multidisciplinary discussion, and the role of interventional radiology in this collaboration has reached the point that they may be considered the fourth pillar in oncology, along with medical, surgical, and radiation oncology.

REFERENCES

1. Livraghi T, Meloni F, Di Stasi M, et al. Sustained complete response and complications rates after radiofrequency ablation of very early hepatocellular carcinoma in cirrhosis: is resection still the treatment of choice? Hepatology 2008; 47(1):82–9.
2. Garden OJ, Rees M, Poston GJ, et al. Guidelines for resection of colorectal cancer liver metastases. Gut 2006;55(Suppl 3):iii1–8.
3. Fong Y, Fortner J, Sun RL, et al. Clinical score for predicting recurrence after hepatic resection for metastatic colorectal cancer: analysis of 1001 consecutive cases. Ann Surg 1999;230(3):309–18 [discussion: 318–21].
4. Choti MA, Sitzmann JV, Tiburi MF, et al. Trends in long-term survival following liver resection for hepatic colorectal metastases. Ann Surg 2002;235(6):759–66.
5. Goldberg RM, Sargent DJ, Morton RF, et al. A randomized controlled trial of fluorouracil plus leucovorin, irinotecan, and oxaliplatin combinations in patients with previously untreated metastatic colorectal cancer. J Clin Oncol 2004;22(1): 23–30.
6. Hurwitz H, Fehrenbacher L, Novotny W, et al. Bevacizumab plus irinotecan, fluorouracil, and leucovorin for metastatic colorectal cancer. N Engl J Med 2004; 350(23):2335–42.
7. Seymour MT, Maughan TS, Ledermann JA, et al. Different strategies of sequential and combination chemotherapy for patients with poor prognosis advanced colorectal cancer (MRC FOCUS): a randomised controlled trial. Lancet 2007; 370(9582):143–52.

8. Pathak S, Jones R, Tang JM, et al. Ablative therapies for colorectal liver metastases: a systematic review. Colorectal Dis 2011;13(9):e252–65.
9. Umeda Y, Matsuda H, Sadamori H, et al. A prognostic model and treatment strategy for intrahepatic recurrence of hepatocellular carcinoma after curative resection. World J Surg 2011;35(1):170–7.
10. Sofocleous CT, Petre EN, Gonen M, et al. CT-guided radiofrequency ablation as a salvage treatment of colorectal cancer hepatic metastases developing after hepatectomy. J Vasc Interv Radiol 2011;22(6):755–61.
11. Erinjeri JP, Fong AJ, Kemeny NE, et al. Timing of administration of bevacizumab chemotherapy affects wound healing after chest wall port placement. Cancer 2011;117(6):1296–301.
12. Sofocleous CT, Nascimento RG, Petrovic LM, et al. Histopathologic and immunohistochemical features of tissue adherent to multitined electrodes after RF ablation of liver malignancies can help predict local tumor progression: initial results. Radiology 2008;249(1):364–74.
13. Solbiati L, Livraghi T, Goldberg SN, et al. Percutaneous radio-frequency ablation of hepatic metastases from colorectal cancer: long-term results in 117 patients. Radiology 2001;221(1):159–66.
14. Gillams AR, Lees WR. Radio-frequency ablation of colorectal liver metastases in 167 patients. Eur Radiol 2004;14(12):2261–7.
15. White TJ, Roy-Choudhury SH, Breen DJ, et al. Percutaneous radiofrequency ablation of colorectal hepatic metastases - initial experience. An adjunct technique to systemic chemotherapy for those with inoperable colorectal hepatic metastases. Dig Surg 2004;21(4):314–20.
16. Feliberti EC, Wagman LD. Radiofrequency ablation of liver metastases from colorectal carcinoma. Cancer Control 2006;13(1):48–51.
17. Hur H, Ko YT, Min BS, et al. Comparative study of resection and radiofrequency ablation in the treatment of solitary colorectal liver metastases. Am J Surg 2009;197(6):728–36.
18. Otto G, Duber C, Hoppe-Lotichius M, et al. Radiofrequency ablation as first-line treatment in patients with early colorectal liver metastases amenable to surgery. Ann Surg 2010;251(5):796–803.
19. Solbiati L, Ahmed M, Cova L, et al. Small liver colorectal metastases treated with percutaneous radiofrequency ablation: local response rate and long-term survival with up to 10-year follow-up. Radiology 2012;265(3):958–68.
20. Oshowo A, Gillams A, Harrison E, et al. Comparison of resection and radiofrequency ablation for treatment of solitary colorectal liver metastases. Br J Surg 2003;90(10):1240–3.
21. Park IJ, Kim HC, Yu CS, et al. Radiofrequency ablation for metachronous liver metastasis from colorectal cancer after curative surgery. Ann Surg Oncol 2008;15(1):227–32.
22. White R, Avital I, Sofocleous C, et al. Rates and patterns of recurrence for percutaneous radiofrequency ablation and open wedge resection for solitary colorectal liver metastasis. J Gastrointest Surg 2007;11(3):256–63.
23. Berber E, Tsinberg M, Tellioglu G, et al. Resection versus laparoscopic radiofrequency thermal ablation of solitary colorectal liver metastasis. J Gastrointest Surg 2008;12(11):1967–72.
24. Gleisner AL, Choti MA, Assumpcao L, et al. Colorectal liver metastases: recurrence and survival following hepatic resection, radiofrequency ablation, and combined resection-radiofrequency ablation. Arch Surg 2008;143(12):1204–12.

25. Kim KH, Yoon YS, Yu CS, et al. Comparative analysis of radiofrequency ablation and surgical resection for colorectal liver metastases. J Korean Surg Soc 2011; 81(1):25–34.
26. Mulier S, Ruers T, Jamart J, et al. Radiofrequency ablation versus resection for resectable colorectal liver metastases: time for a randomized trial? An update. Dig Surg 2008;25(6):445–60.
27. de Baere T, Elias D, Dromain C, et al. Radiofrequency ablation of 100 hepatic metastases with a mean follow-up of more than 1 year. AJR Am J Roentgenol 2000;175(6):1619–25.
28. Berber E, Pelley R, Siperstein AE. Predictors of survival after radiofrequency thermal ablation of colorectal cancer metastases to the liver: a prospective study. J Clin Oncol 2005;23(7):1358–64.
29. Ruers T, Punt C, Van Coevorden F, et al. Radiofrequency ablation combined with systemic treatment versus systemic treatment alone in patients with non-resectable colorectal liver metastases: a randomized EORTC Intergroup phase II study (EORTC 40004). Ann Oncol 2012;23(10):2619–26.
30. Pawlik TM, Tanabe KK. Radiofrequency ablation for primary and metastatic liver tumors. Cancer Treat Res 2001;109:247–67.
31. Kuvshinoff BW, Ota DM. Radiofrequency ablation of liver tumors: influence of technique and tumor size. Surgery 2002;132(4):605–11 [discussion: 611–2].
32. Kei SK, Rhim H, Choi D, et al. Local tumor progression after radiofrequency ablation of liver tumors: analysis of morphologic pattern and site of recurrence. AJR Am J Roentgenol 2008;190(6):1544–51.
33. Rossi S, Garbagnati F, Lencioni R, et al. Percutaneous radio-frequency thermal ablation of nonresectable hepatocellular carcinoma after occlusion of tumor blood supply. Radiology 2000;217(1):119–26.
34. Mulier S, Ni Y, Jamart J, et al. Radiofrequency ablation versus resection for resectable colorectal liver metastases: time for a randomized trial? Ann Surg Oncol 2008;15(1):144–57.
35. Livraghi T, Solbiati L, Meloni F, et al. Percutaneous radiofrequency ablation of liver metastases in potential candidates for resection: the "test-of-time approach". Cancer 2003;97(12):3027–35.
36. Kim YS, Rhim H, Cho OK, et al. Intrahepatic recurrence after percutaneous radiofrequency ablation of hepatocellular carcinoma: analysis of the pattern and risk factors. Eur J Radiol 2006;59(3):432–41.
37. Ayav A, Germain A, Marchal F, et al. Radiofrequency ablation of unresectable liver tumors: factors associated with incomplete ablation or local recurrence. Am J Surg 2010;200(4):435–9.
38. Mulier S, Ni Y, Jamart J, et al. Local recurrence after hepatic radiofrequency coagulation: multivariate meta-analysis and review of contributing factors. Ann Surg Oncol 2005;242:158–71.
39. Nakazawa T, Kokubu S, Shibuya A, et al. Radiofrequency ablation of hepatocellular carcinoma: correlation between local tumor progression after ablation and ablative margin. AJR Am J Roentgenol 2007;188(2):480–8.
40. Lu DS, Raman SS, Limanond P, et al. Influence of large peritumoral vessels on outcome of radiofrequency ablation of liver tumors. J Vasc Interv Radiol 2003; 14(10):1267–74.
41. de Jong MC, Pulitano C, Ribero D, et al. Rates and patterns of recurrence following curative intent surgery for colorectal liver metastasis: an international multi-institutional analysis of 1669 patients. Ann Surg 2009;250(3):440–8.

42. Kim YS, Lee WJ, Rhim H, et al. The minimal ablative margin of radiofrequency ablation of hepatocellular carcinoma (> 2 and < 5 cm) needed to prevent local tumor progression: 3D quantitative assessment using CT image fusion. AJR Am J Roentgenol 2010;195(3):758–65.

43. Liu CH, Arellano RS, Uppot RN, et al. Radiofrequency ablation of hepatic tumours: effect of post-ablation margin on local tumour progression. Eur Radiol 2010;20(4):877–85.

44. Wang X, Sofocleous CT, Erinjeri JP, et al. Margin size is an independent predictor of local tumor progression after ablation of colon cancer liver metastases. Cardiovasc Intervent Radiol 2012;36:166–75.

45. Seifert JK, Springer A, Baier P, et al. Liver resection or cryotherapy for colorectal liver metastases: a prospective case control study. Int J Colorectal Dis 2005; 20(6):507–20.

46. Niu R, Yan TD, Zhu JC, et al. Recurrence and survival outcomes after hepatic resection with or without cryotherapy for liver metastases from colorectal carcinoma. Ann Surg Oncol 2007;14(7):2078–87.

47. Ng KM, Chua TC, Saxena A, et al. Two decades of experience with hepatic cryotherapy for advanced colorectal metastases. Ann Surg Oncol 2012;19(4):1276–83.

48. Groeschl RT, Pilgrim CH, Hanna EM, et al. Microwave ablation for hepatic malignancies: a multiinstitutional analysis. Ann Surg 2013;259:1195–200.

49. Tanaka K, Shimada H, Nagano Y, et al. Outcome after hepatic resection versus combined resection and microwave ablation for multiple bilobar colorectal metastases to the liver. Surgery 2006;139(2):263–73.

50. Ogata Y, Uchida S, Hisaka T, et al. Intraoperative thermal ablation therapy for small colorectal metastases to the liver. Hepatogastroenterology 2008; 55(82–83):550–6.

51. Shibata T, Niinobu T, Ogata N, et al. Microwave coagulation therapy for multiple hepatic metastases from colorectal carcinoma. Cancer 2000;89(2):276–84.

52. Cannon R, Ellis S, Hayes D, et al. Safety and early efficacy of irreversible electroporation for hepatic tumors in proximity to vital structures. J Surg Oncol 2013; 107(5):544–9.

53. Thomson KR, Cheung W, Ellis SJ, et al. Investigation of the safety of irreversible electroporation in humans. J Vasc Interv Radiol 2011;22(5):611–21.

54. Silk MT, Wimmer T, Lee KS, et al. Percutaneous ablation of peribiliary tumors with irreversible electroporation. J Vasc Interv Radiol 2014;25(1):112–8.

55. Kingham TP, Karkar AM, D'Angelica MI, et al. Ablation of perivascular hepatic malignant tumors with irreversible electroporation. J Am Coll Surg 2012; 215(3):379–87.

56. de Baere T, Deschamps F. Arterial therapies of colorectal cancer metastases to the liver. Abdom Imaging 2011;36(6):661–70.

57. Kemeny NE, Melendez FD, Capanu M, et al. Conversion to resectability using hepatic artery infusion plus systemic chemotherapy for the treatment of unresectable liver metastases from colorectal carcinoma. J Clin Oncol 2009; 27(21):3465–71.

58. Cohen AD, Kemeny NE. An update on hepatic arterial infusion chemotherapy for colorectal cancer. Oncologist 2003;8(6):553–66.

59. Kemeny M. Hepatic artery infusion of chemotherapy as a treatment for hepatic metastases from colorectal cancer. Cancer J 2002;8(Suppl 1):S82–8.

60. Ganeshan A, Upponi S, Hon LQ, et al. Hepatic arterial infusion of chemotherapy: the role of diagnostic and interventional radiology. Ann Oncol 2008;19(5): 847–51.

61. Nakakuma K, Tashiro S, Hiraoka T, et al. Hepatocellular carcinoma and metastatic cancer detected by iodized oil. Radiology 1985;154(1):15–7.

62. Konno T, Maeda H, Iwai K, et al. Selective targeting of anticancer drug and simultaneous image enhancement in solid tumors by arterially administered lipid contrast medium. Cancer 1984;54(11):2367–74.

63. de Baere T, Dufaux J, Roche A, et al. Circulatory alterations induced by intra-arterial injection of iodized oil and emulsions of iodized oil and doxorubicin: experimental study. Radiology 1995;194(1):165–70.

64. Egawa H, Maki A, Mori K, et al. Effects of intra-arterial chemotherapy with a new lipophilic anticancer agent, estradiol-chlorambucil (KM2210), dissolved in lipiodol on experimental liver tumor in rats. J Surg Oncol 1990;44(2): 109–14.

65. Kruskal JB, Hlatky L, Hahnfeldt P, et al. In vivo and in vitro analysis of the effectiveness of doxorubicin combined with temporary arterial occlusion in liver tumors. J Vasc Interv Radiol 1993;4(6):741–7.

66. Albert M, Kiefer MV, Sun W, et al. Chemoembolization of colorectal liver metastases with cisplatin, doxorubicin, mitomycin C, ethiodol, and polyvinyl alcohol. Cancer 2011;117(2):343–52.

67. Vogl TJ, Gruber T, Balzer JO, et al. Repeated transarterial chemoembolization in the treatment of liver metastases of colorectal cancer: prospective study. Radiology 2009;250(1):281–9.

68. Taylor RR, Tang Y, Gonzalez MV, et al. Irinotecan drug eluting beads for use in chemoembolization: in vitro and in vivo evaluation of drug release properties. Eur J Pharm Sci 2007;30(1):7–14.

69. Fiorentini G, Aliberti C, Tilli M, et al. Intra-arterial infusion of irinotecan-loaded drug-eluting beads (DEBIRI) versus intravenous therapy (FOLFIRI) for hepatic metastases from colorectal cancer: final results of a phase III study. Anticancer Res 2012;32(4):1387–95.

70. Martin RC, Joshi J, Robbins K, et al. Hepatic intra-arterial injection of drug-eluting bead, irinotecan (DEBIRI) in unresectable colorectal liver metastases refractory to systemic chemotherapy: results of multi-institutional study. Ann Surg Oncol 2011;18(1):192–8.

71. Hong K, McBride JD, Georgiades CS, et al. Salvage therapy for liver-dominant colorectal metastatic adenocarcinoma: comparison between transcatheter arterial chemoembolization versus yttrium-90 radioembolization. J Vasc Interv Radiol 2009;20(3):360–7.

72. Martin RC, Howard J, Tomalty D, et al. Toxicity of irinotecan-eluting beads in the treatment of hepatic malignancies: results of a multi-institutional registry. Cardiovasc Intervent Radiol 2010;33(5):960–6.

73. Russell AH, Clyde C, Wasserman TH, et al. Accelerated hyperfractionated hepatic irradiation in the management of patients with liver metastases: results of the RTOG dose escalating protocol. Int J Radiat Oncol Biol Phys 1993; 27(1):117–23.

74. Emami B, Lyman J, Brown A, et al. Tolerance of normal tissue to therapeutic irradiation. Int J Radiat Oncol Biol Phys 1991;21(1):109–22.

75. Dawson LA, McGinn CJ, Normolle D, et al. Escalated focal liver radiation and concurrent hepatic artery fluorodeoxyuridine for unresectable intrahepatic malignancies. J Clin Oncol 2000;18(11):2210–8.

76. Kennedy AS, Nutting C, Coldwell D, et al. Pathologic response and microdosimetry of (90)Y microspheres in man: review of four explanted whole livers. Int J Radiat Oncol Biol Phys 2004;60(5):1552–63.

77. Sofocleous CT, Garcia AR, Pandit-Taskar N, et al. Phase I trial of selective internal radiation therapy for chemorefractory colorectal cancer liver metastases progressing after hepatic arterial pump and systemic chemotherapy. Clin Colorectal Cancer 2013;13:27–36.

78. Kennedy AS, Coldwell D, Nutting C, et al. Resin ^{90}Y-microsphere brachytherapy for unresectable colorectal liver metastases: modern USA experience. Int J Radiat Oncol Biol Phys 2006;65(2):412–25.

79. Jakobs TF, Hoffmann RT, Dehm K, et al. Hepatic yttrium-90 radioembolization of chemotherapy-refractory colorectal cancer liver metastases. J Vasc Interv Radiol 2008;19(8):1187–95.

80. Vente MA, Wondergem M, van der Tweel I, et al. Yttrium-90 microsphere radioembolization for the treatment of liver malignancies: a structured meta-analysis. Eur Radiol 2009;19(4):951–9.

81. Cosimelli M, Golfieri R, Cagol PP, et al. Multi-centre phase II clinical trial of yttrium-90 resin microspheres alone in unresectable, chemotherapy refractory colorectal liver metastases. Br J Cancer 2010;103(3):324–31.

82. Van Hazel G, Blackwell A, Anderson J, et al. Randomised phase 2 trial of SIR-Spheres plus fluorouracil/leucovorin chemotherapy versus fluorouracil/leucovorin chemotherapy alone in advanced colorectal cancer. J Surg Oncol 2004; 88(2):78–85.

83. Hendlisz A, Van den Eynde M, Peeters M, et al. Phase III trial comparing protracted intravenous fluorouracil infusion alone or with yttrium-90 resin microspheres radioembolization for liver-limited metastatic colorectal cancer refractory to standard chemotherapy. J Clin Oncol 2010;28(23):3687–94.

84. Nicolay NH, Berry DP, Sharma RA. Liver metastases from colorectal cancer: radioembolization with systemic therapy. Nat Rev Clin Oncol 2009;6(12): 687–97.

85. Watanabe K, Nagai K, Kobayashi A, et al. Factors influencing survival after complete resection of pulmonary metastases from colorectal cancer. Br J Surg 2009; 96(9):1058–65.

86. Long-term results of lung metastasectomy: prognostic analyses based on 5206 cases. The International Registry of Lung Metastases. J Thorac Cardiovasc Surg 1997;113(1):37–49.

87. Mori M, Tomoda H, Ishida T, et al. Surgical resection of pulmonary metastases from colorectal adenocarcinoma. Special reference to repeated pulmonary resections. Arch Surg 1991;126(10):1297–301 [discussion: 1302].

88. Saito Y, Omiya H, Kohno K, et al. Pulmonary metastasectomy for 165 patients with colorectal carcinoma: a prognostic assessment. J Thorac Cardiovasc Surg 2002;124(5):1007–13.

89. Li WH, Peng JJ, Xiang JQ, et al. Oncological outcome of unresectable lung metastases without extrapulmonary metastases in colorectal cancer. World J Gastroenterol 2010;16(26):3318–24.

90. Lencioni R, Crocetti L, Cioni R, et al. Response to radiofrequency ablation of pulmonary tumours: a prospective, intention-to-treat, multicentre clinical trial (the RAPTURE study). Lancet Oncol 2008;9(7):621–8.

91. Yan TD, King J, Sjarif A, et al. Treatment failure after percutaneous radiofrequency ablation for nonsurgical candidates with pulmonary metastases from colorectal carcinoma. Ann Surg Oncol 2007;14(5):1718–26.

92. Yamakado K, Hase S, Matsuoka T, et al. Radiofrequency ablation for the treatment of unresectable lung metastases in patients with colorectal cancer: a multicenter study in Japan. J Vasc Interv Radiol 2007;18(3):393–8.

93. Hiraki T, Gobara H, Iishi T, et al. Percutaneous radiofrequency ablation for pulmonary metastases from colorectal cancer: midterm results in 27 patients. J Vasc Interv Radiol 2007;18(10):1264–9.
94. Petre EN, Jia X, Thornton RH, et al. Treatment of pulmonary colorectal metastases by radiofrequency ablation. Clin Colorectal Cancer 2013;12(1):37–44.
95. Gillams A, Khan Z, Osborn P, et al. Survival after radiofrequency ablation in 122 patients with inoperable colorectal lung metastases. Cardiovasc Intervent Radiol 2013;36(3):724–30.
96. Yamakado K, Inoue Y, Takao M, et al. Long-term results of radiofrequency ablation in colorectal lung metastases: single center experience. Oncol Rep 2009; 22(4):885–91.
97. Vogl TJ, Naguib NN, Gruber-Rouh T, et al. Microwave ablation therapy: clinical utility in treatment of pulmonary metastases. Radiology 2011;261(2):643–51.
98. Khuri SF, Henderson WG, DePalma RG, et al. Determinants of long-term survival after major surgery and the adverse effect of postoperative complications. Ann Surg 2005;242(3):326–41 [discussion: 341–3].
99. Hiromichi I, Chandrakanth A, Gonen M, et al. Effect of postoperative morbidity on long-term survival after hepatic resection for metastatic CRC. Ann Surg 2008;247(6):994–1002.
100. Gray B, Van Hazel G, Hope M, et al. Randomised trial of SIR-Spheres plus chemotherapy vs. chemotherapy alone for treating patients with liver metastases from primary large bowel cancer. Ann Oncol 2001;12(12):1711–20.

Nonoperative Management of Rectal Cancer: Identifying the Ideal Patients

Angelita Habr-Gama, MD, PhD[a,b,*],
Guilherme Pagin São Julião, MD[a], Rodrigo O. Perez, MD, PhD[a,c]

KEYWORDS

- Rectal cancer • Neoadjuvant chemoradiation therapy • Complete clinical response
- Watch and wait

KEY POINTS

- If you are considering a watch-and-wait policy for patients with a complete clinical response (cCR), you should consider treating cT2N0 low rectal tumors with neoadjuvant chemoradiation.
- The best tool to assess cCR is digital rectal examination and endoscopy. Endoscopic biopsy results may be misleading.
- Radiological imaging does not diagnose cCR; it just confirms it. In the absence of cCR, do not look for radiological evidence to support nonoperative management.
- Local excision (full excisional biopsy) is a good tool to assess primary tumor response in patients with near cCR and radiological imaging showing ycT0-2N0.

 Videos of an endoscopic view of complete clinical response and a full-thickness local excision accompany this article at http://www.hemonc.theclinics.com/

INTRODUCTION

Rectal cancer management has become increasingly complex over the last few decades.[1] The widespread use of neoadjuvant therapies has introduced a new variable, tumor response, which may dramatically change the ultimate surgical decision from

[a] Angelita and Joaquim Gama Institute, Rua Manoel da Nóbrega 1564, Paraiso, São Paulo 04001-005, Brazil; [b] University of São Paulo School of Medicine, Rua Manoel da Nóbrega 1564, Paraiso, São Paulo 04001-005, Brazil; [c] Colorectal Surgery Division, Department of Gastroenterology, University of São Paulo School of Medicine, Rua Manoel da Nóbrega 1564, Paraiso, São Paulo 04001-005, Brazil
* Corresponding author. University of São Paulo School of Medicine, Rua Manoel da Nóbrega 1564, Paraiso, São Paulo 04001-005, Brazil.
E-mail address: gamange@uol.com.br

Hematol Oncol Clin N Am 29 (2015) 135–151
http://dx.doi.org/10.1016/j.hoc.2014.09.004
0889-8588/15/$ – see front matter © 2015 Elsevier Inc. All rights reserved.

radical surgery to local excision, transanal endoscopic microsurgery (TEM), or even no surgery at all. In this setting, surgeons have to consider many aspects of the disease before deciding on a definitive treatment approach.

INDICATIONS FOR NEOADJUVANT THERAPY

Classic indications for neoadjuvant therapy in rectal cancer are mostly derived from randomized controlled studies that showed a local control benefit among patients with cT3-4 or cN+ tumors treated with radiation or chemoradiation (CRT), followed by radical surgery.[2,3] However, recent updates with a longer follow-up of these same cohorts suggest that the benefits in local disease control following neoadjuvant CRT and radical surgery are marginal or even outweighed by treatment-related toxicities.[4–6] Therefore, except for circumferential margin positivity, local control is not expected to be significantly increased with the use of neoadjuvant CRT provided appropriate total mesorectal excision is performed, even for cT3 or cN+ disease (**Box 1**).

On the other hand, neoadjuvant radiation alone, CRT, or even chemotherapy alone may lead to significant tumor regression resulting in[7,8]

- Downsizing (significant changes in tumor size)
- Downstaging (depth of penetration)
- Nodal sterilization
- Pathologic complete response (pCR)

Not only does this latter group of patients with pCR have improved oncological outcomes but also the opportunity of being spared from radical surgery and its associated immediate morbidity, mortality, functional disorders, and need for stomas.[9–11]

The problem is that if you give neoadjuvant therapy only for advanced stage disease, very few patients will develop a complete tumor response (up to 24%).[9] However, neoadjuvant therapy may be extremely useful for the selection of those patients who may avoid a radical operation and, thus, may be used more effectively if more widely adopted to include patients with earlier disease stages. If earlier disease stages are offered this treatment strategy (including cT2N0), complete response may develop more frequently, reaching up to 44% of patients, and would allow more patients to benefit from avoiding radical surgery and associated morbidities.[12–16]

In a recent study of patients with cT2N0 rectal cancer undergoing CRT followed by full-thickness local excision (FTLE), pCR in the primary tumor (ypT0) was observed in 44% of patients, suggesting that a significant proportion of these patients with an earlier disease stage may benefit the most from neoadjuvant CRT.[14]

Box 1
Potential long-term detrimental consequences from radiation therapy

- Increased rates of second primary cancers
- Small-bowel obstruction
- Chronic abdominal pain

Data from Birgisson H, Pahlman L, Gunnarsson U, et al. Occurrence of second cancers in patients treated with radiotherapy for rectal cancer. J Clin Oncol 2005;23:6126–31; and Birgisson H, Pahlman L, Gunnarsson U, et al. Adverse effects of preoperative radiation therapy for rectal cancer: long-term follow-up of the Swedish Rectal Cancer Trial. J Clin Oncol 2005;23:8697–705.

TYPES OF NEOADJUVANT THERAPY

Considering neoadjuvant therapy will be used for the purpose of tailoring surgical therapy for patients based on the tumor response, strategies associated with significant tumor regression are preferred.[1] Therefore, combined association of chemotherapy and radiation (ie, long-course with hyperfractionated radiation therapy (RT) doses) has been shown to result in greater tumor regression rates and an increased chance of a complete response.[7,13] In contrast, short-course RT alone may only lead to significant tumor regression if longer intervals between RT completion and assessment of the response are allowed.[17] The standard days to 1-week interval will lead to virtually no chance of developing a pCR.[18]

Finally, even though most studies have dealt with radiation or CRT therapies in the neoadjuvant setting, there is a suggestion that chemotherapy alone could provide similar outcomes in terms of rates of pathologic response and, therefore, sparing patients from potentially unnecessary radiation-related toxicities.[8] In fact, a regimen with radiation and an increased number of cycles of chemotherapy has resulted in surprisingly high rates of complete tumor regression (51% complete clinical response [cCR]). It has been the authors' practice to offer patients this extended CRT regimen, especially considering that the chances of having a complete response are higher (**Fig. 1**).[19,20]

ASSESSING TUMOR RESPONSE
Why?

The rationale for assessing the tumor response after neoadjuvant therapy is to define the final treatment strategy based on the current status of the tumor, that is, after therapy.

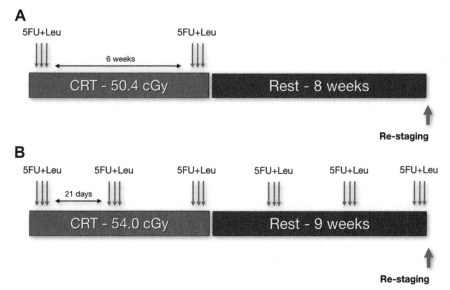

Fig. 1. Neoadjuvant CRT regimen. (*A*) Standard long-course CRT regimen. (*B*) Extended CRT regimen with consolidation chemotherapy. 5FU, 5-fluorouracil. Leu, Leucovorin. (*Data from* Habr-Gama A, Perez RO, Sabbaga J, et al. Increasing the rates of complete response to neoadjuvant chemoradiotherapy for distal rectal cancer: results of a prospective study using additional chemotherapy during the resting period. Dis Colon Rectum 2009;52:1927–34.)

In a significant proportion of patients undergoing neoadjuvant CRT, complete tumor regression may develop. The problem is that most of the time radical surgery is required to appropriately confirm the presence of a pCR. In an effort to spare patients from potentially unnecessary surgery, colorectal surgeons have attempted to assess the tumor response in order to estimate the pathologic response by clinical, endoscopic, and radiological means.

In this setting, the term cCR has been used for patients with no clinical evidence of residual cancer after neoadjuvant therapy.

It has been suggested that patients with cCR (*using very stringent criteria*) might be offered no immediate radical surgery. Instead, a strict surveillance program, also know as the *watch-and-wait strategy*, with frequent visits to the colorectal surgeon and the use of multiple staging modalities could possibly provide a safe follow-up. Initial studies trying to estimate the accuracy of clinical assessment in predicting pCR were disappointing.[21] However, more recent studies have shown that clinical assessment can accurately detect pCR when stringent criteria are used.[22]

When?

Intervals between CRT completion and the assessment of response may also be relevant. Studies suggest that longer intervals are associated with higher pCR rates.[23–25] Initially 2 weeks was used, then 6 weeks, and now intervals as long as 12 weeks are considered.[26] There are ongoing randomized studies to address these issues that will provide us further information on the ideal interval between CRT and the assessment of response. There is a chance, however, that intervals will need to be tailored or individualized for each patient, as tumors may respond differently as a function of time to treatment.[27] In a recent study using sequential PET/computed tomography (CT) imaging, patients showed a significant decrease in tumor metabolism between baseline and 6 weeks from standard CRT, estimated by maximum standard uptake value (SUV-max) values. However, between 6 and 12 weeks there were 2 subgroups of tumor metabolism profiles. Although half of the patients developed a further decrease in standard uptake value (SUV) between 6 and 12 weeks, the remaining half developed an increase in SUV, suggesting tumor repopulation (**Fig. 2**).[27] It will be interesting to see these metabolism profiles after newer and more intensive CRT regimens.

It has been the authors' practice since 1991, from the beginning of their experience with CRT for distal rectal cancer, to assess the tumor response at least 8 weeks from CRT completion.[28] More recently, however, longer intervals (up to 12 weeks) have been used for most patients.

How?

Response assessment always begins with the characterization of symptoms. Symptomatic patients rarely have complete tumor regression, even though this feature has very low specificity. Digital rectal examination (DRE) is perhaps one of the most relevant tools in tumor response assessment. There is currently no single diagnostic tool that can replace the information given by DRE. Frequently, irregularities of the rectal wall are better felt than seen and should be considered as highly suspicious for residual cancer. No patient is considered for a nonoperative approach in the presence of rectal wall irregularities, mass, ulceration, or stenosis. A cCR is defined as the absence of any irregularity of the rectal wall. The area can be thickened and firm; but to be considered a cCR, the surface has to be regular and smooth.[29]

Endoscopic assessment is also very important (**Box 2**). The presence of any ulceration or mucosal irregularity missed on DRE should prompt additional investigations and usually rules out a cCR (**Fig. 3**). During flexible or rigid proctoscopy, biopsies

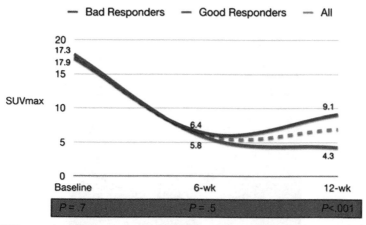

Fig. 2. SUVmax values from sequential PET/CT for patients with rectal cancer, before CRT, 6 weeks after CRT, and 12 weeks after CRT. (*Data from* Perez RO, Habr-Gama A, Sao Juliao GP, et al. Optimal timing for assessment of tumor response to neoadjuvant chemoradiation in patients with rectal cancer: do all patients benefit from waiting longer than 6 weeks? Int J Radiat Oncol Biol Phys 2012;84:1159–65.)

are frequently considered for the assessment of response. However, the results of endoscopic biopsies should be interpreted with caution (**Box 3**).

LOCAL EXCISION OF THE TUMOR SITE

For patients with small residual lesions, the authors usually offer a FTLE, preferably with the use of TEM as a diagnostic procedure (Video 2)

- Small lesions (≤3 cm)
- Low lesions, otherwise candidate for abdominal-perineal excision (APE) or a coloanal intersphincteric resection
- No evidence of mesorectal dissemination by imaging studies

It has been the authors' policy to offer strict follow-up to patients with a final pathologic specimen showing ypT0 after this diagnostic FTLE because the risk of lymph node metastases among these patients has been shown to be very low in the setting of neoadjuvant CRT and long intervals (≥8 weeks). This finding is already true for unselected patients with ypT0, whereby the risk of nodal metastases is well less than 10% and in most cases less than 5%.[32–34] However, with the significant

---

Box 2
Frequent endoscopic findings consistent with cCR (Video 1)

- No residual mass, ulceration or stenosis
- Whitening of the mucosa
- Telangiectasias

Data from Habr-Gama A, Perez RO, Wynn G, et al. Complete clinical response after neoadjuvant chemoradiation therapy for distal rectal cancer: characterization of clinical and endoscopic findings for standardization. Dis Colon Rectum 2010;53:1692–8.

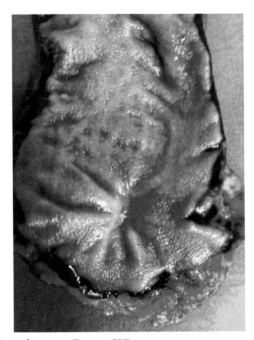

Fig. 3. Residual lesion after neoadjuvant CRT.

improvements in radiological imaging, particularly with high-resolution magnetic resonance (MR) with the use of diffusion-weighted series and lymphotropic agents, the selection of patients with ycT0N0 is expected to further improve (**Box 4**).[35]

Equally challenging patients are those with intermediate residual cancers: ypT1 or early ypT2 (restricted to the superficial muscular layer) cancers without lymphovascular invasion or other unfavorable pathologic features, particularly among patients that would otherwise be candidates for APE or coloanal anastomosis. In the presence of negative margins (≥5 mm), it has been the authors' policy to follow up these patients without immediate radical surgery. This strategy of offering patients with small superficial residual cancers, radiologically staged as ycN0, a local procedure is quite appealing. However, there are at least 2 main drawbacks to this treatment strategy:

- Healing of the rectal defects determined by FTLE after neoadjuvant CRT are quite challenging and painful, particularly those closer to anal verge (**Fig. 5**).[36,37]

Box 3
Endoscopic biopsies for suspected cCR

A recent study analyzed the presence of residual cancer among different layers of the rectal wall. Curiously, the presence of cancer cells within deeper layers of the rectum was frequently observed among tumors without cancer at the mucosal level. Therefore, endoscopic mucosal biopsies would lead to false-negative results in a significant amount of these patients.[30] In a review of patients with significant tumor regression after neoadjuvant CRT managed by surgical resection, preoperative biopsies showed a negative predictive value of endoscopic biopsies was as low as 21%.[31] If there is clinical evidence (DRE and endoscopic) of a cCR, forceps biopsies should be interpreted with caution because a negative biopsy cannot rule out microscopic residual cancer.[31]

Box 4
Unfavorable pathologic findings after FTLE as excisional biopsy

- YpT3
- Lymphovascular invasion (**Fig. 4**)
- Positive resection margins

- Sphincter preservation may be compromised after performance of FTLE in this setting.

A few studies have addressed this issue and reported that patients requiring radical resection after FTLE almost always ended up with an APE, even though they were originally considered candidates for a sphincter-preserving procedure.[38,39] Both of these issues should be kept in mind when offering patients diagnostic or therapeutic local excision after partial response (**Box 5**).

RADIOLOGICAL IMAGING

Radiological assessment of response is of paramount importance to appropriately select patients for an alternative treatment strategy, such as the watch-and-wait approach, following a cCR. As a matter of fact, the developments in radiological imaging, including both PET/CT and MR, have been quite significant. Proper MRI with the use of diffusion-weighted techniques are now used routinely for the assessment of response in these patients.[40] Currently, the authors would only consider a true complete responder if there is no evidence of disease on clinical and endoscopic examination and

- Low-signal-intensity area replacing the area of the previous tumor in MR (**Fig. 6**)
- No detectable abnormalities in standard MR
- Absence of restriction to diffusion in diffusion-weighted MR[40]

Some investigators have attempted to estimate tumor regression grades (as described for pathologic assessment)[41] by standard MRI.[42] In the authors' previously

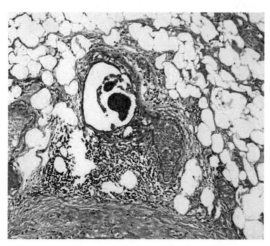

Fig. 4. Lymphovascular invasion. Hematoloxilin and Eosin, original magnification ×400.

142

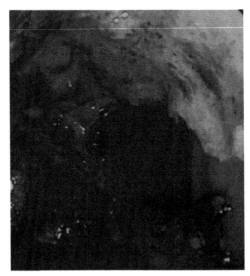

Fig. 5. Wound dehiscence after FTLE.

Box 5
Why not offer patients with a cCR transanal local excision for the histologic confirmation of ypT0?

As mentioned earlier, healing of local excision defects following neoadjuvant CRT is not as simple as after local excision alone. The rates of wound dehiscence may be quite significant. In this setting, not only is pain an issue but also significant scarring following delayed healing may develop which will make patient follow-up even more difficult. Even though ypT0 may be associated with a lower risk of local failures, the risk is not zero and patients still require appropriate follow-up. Distinction between local recurrence in a rectal wall following wound dehiscence after a local excision with or without rectal stenosis may be quite challenging. Therefore, the authors think that follow-up is considerably facilitated by preservation of rectal wall integrity with the watch-and-wait approach allowing for earlier detection of eventual recurrences in addition to superior functional outcomes.

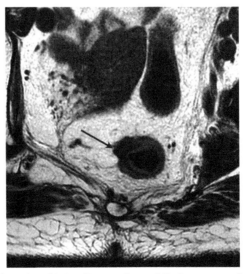

Fig. 6. MR showing low signal intensity area (*arrow*) that correspond to fibrosis and cCR.

reported experiences with this watch-and-wait treatment strategy, MRI was not available to a significant proportion of patients.[43] Therefore, there is a hope that incorporation of these findings for the selection of patients with cCR will significantly impact the outcomes of the watch-and-wait strategy (**Box 6**). The presence of mixed signal intensity (**Fig. 7**) within the area of the previous cancer should raise a suspicion of an incomplete clinical response. In addition to the assessment of the rectal wall, the mesorectum is also at risk for the presence of residual cancer despite complete primary regression (ypT0N1). Therefore, MRI should also provide the colorectal surgeon with information regarding possible mesorectal (or even lateral node) involvement regardless of the primary tumor response (**Box 7, Fig. 8**). An alternative to MR is endorectal ultrasound that can also offer good accuracy staging of rectal cancer after neoadjuvant CRT (**Fig. 9**).[44,45]

Molecular imaging may also play a role in the assessment of tumor response. PET/CT has been used for the assessment of tumor response to neoadjuvant CRT therapy.[12,46] In addition to the visual identification of fluoro-2-deoxy-D-glucose (FDG) uptake within the area of the rectal wall harboring the tumor or within the mesorectum, PET/CT allows the estimation of the metabolism profile. Standard uptake values are direct estimations of tissue metabolism and may be used for the distinction of residual inflammatory changes and residual cancer.

The authors have used PET/CT to distinguish between complete and incomplete responses in the setting of a prospective study with acceptable overall accuracy (85%). However, the authors consider PET/CT not appropriate for routine use for this purpose, mainly because of the increased cost and need for multiple studies with significant radiation exposure.[12] Instead, the use of this molecular imaging modality should perhaps be considered for patients with significant discordant results between studies, particularly between clinical and radiological findings (**Box 8, Fig. 10**).

CARCINOEMBRYONIC ANTIGEN

Pretreatment carcinoembryonic antigen (CEA) levels have been shown to be predictors of the response to neoadjuvant CRT and ultimately survival.[41,47] Posttreatment CEA levels are also relevant, and normal levels after CRT have been associated with increased cCR rates.[48] Abnormal CEA levels before or after CRT should raise the suspicion of an incomplete response to CRT and/or metastatic dissemination (**Box 9**).[49]

SUMMARY PEARLS
Final Decision Management

1. Patients are usually assessed for tumor response to neoadjuvant CRT at least 8 to 12 weeks from treatment completion.

Box 6
Patterns low-signal intensity compatible with cCR

- Minimal fibrosis
- Transmural fibrosis
- Irregular fibrosis

Data from Lambregts DM, Maas M, Bakers FC, et al. Long-term follow-up features on rectal MRI during a wait-and-see approach after a clinical complete response in patients with rectal cancer treated with chemoradiotherapy. Dis Colon Rectum 2011;54:1521–8.

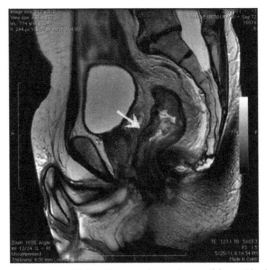

Fig. 7. MR showing mixed signal intensity area (*arrow*), possible residual tumor.

Box 7
Complete radiological response: MR

- Low signal in the rectal wall = fibrosis
- Normal or absent lymph node

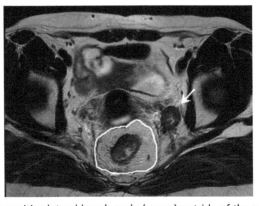

Fig. 8. MR showing positive lateral lymph node (*arrow*) outside of the mesorectum (circle).

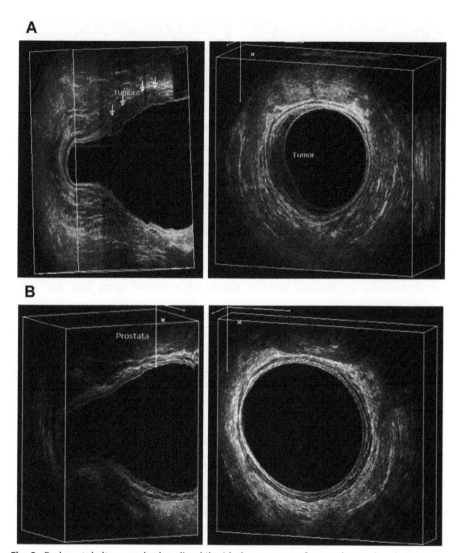

Fig. 9. Endorectal ultrasound at baseline (*A*) with the presence of tumor (*arrows*) and at reassessment with complete response showing no detectable abnormality (*B*).

Box 8
PET/CT predicting residual cancer
Measurement of SUV in 2 different intervals from FDG injection is routinely performed (at 1 and 3 hours) and allows 2 distinct patterns (dual time) of metabolism. Increases in SUVs (between 1 and 3 hours) suggest the presence of residual cancer, whereas decreases suggest inflammatory or fibrotic changes.[27]

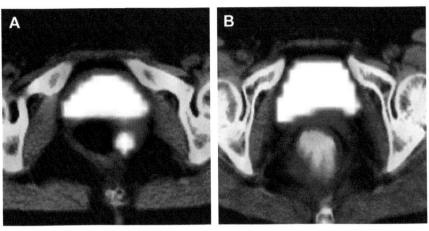

Fig. 10. PET/CT baseline (*A*) and at reassessment with complete response (*B*).

2. Assessment
   - Clinical and endoscopic features should be assessed using DRE and rigid proctoscopy.
   - Flexible proctoscopy is used solely for video documentation.
   - CEA levels should be normal both before and after treatment, otherwise additional studies are strongly recommended.
   - MR should be performed for 2 purposes:
     - Confirmation of findings consistent with a complete response within the rectal wall
     - Confirmation of the absence of dissemination to mesorectal or lateral nodes

Usually, MR with diffusion-weighted series is sufficient for most cases. In patients with an incomplete clinical response caused by subtle mucosal irregularities, radiological staging that indicates complete response and a normal CEA (before and after CRT), transanal local excision (preferably using TEM) may be used primarily as a diagnostic procedure. In patients with a cCR but with radiological evidence of residual disease on MR or abnormal CEA levels (before or after treatment), PET/CT may be a useful assessment tool. A normal PET/CT may still allow consideration of a nonoperative approach in select cases after discussion with patients. Abnormal PET/CT in this setting should be viewed as highly suspicious for residual cancer. Incomplete clinical response (gross residual cancer or ulceration) should prompt restaging to allow proper determination of final surgical approach but never to suggest a nonoperative approach.

Patients suspected for a cCR are closely followed and reassessed for tumor response every 1 to 2 months for the first year, every 3 months for the second year, and every 6 months thereafter. If initial radiological assessment of response is normal (MR) or consistent with a complete response, radiological reassessment may be performed at 6 months from the initial assessment (**Box 10**).

Box 9
Abnormal CEA after neoadjuvant CRT

Abnormal CEA levels should lead to a more liberal use of PET/CT imaging for the assessment of tumor response because it may also allow the detection of unsuspected metastatic disease in addition to the diagnosis of incomplete response.

> **Box 10**
> **Additional therapy**
>
> Until now, patients with a cCR have not been offered adjuvant systemic therapy of any kind following nonoperative management. However, the risk of systemic recurrence among these patients is still significant and may ultimately justify its use in selected patients according to baseline radiological features, such as nodal positivity. Therefore, even though high-risk patients (cT3N+ at baseline staging) may still be considered for a nonoperative approach after a cCR following CRT, adjuvant systemic chemotherapy may prove to be beneficial. Even though this may sound appropriate, it warrants further investigation in properly designed prospective studies.

LOCAL RECURRENCE AND SALVAGE

Local recurrence after no immediate surgery following a cCR may develop at any time during the follow-up of these patients. Even though there is no accepted standard definition of recurrence in terms of timing after CRT, it has been the authors' policy to consider early recurrences developing within the initial 12 months of follow-up as early tumor regrowths.[16] Early tumor regrowths have been reported in up to 19% of patients undergoing standard CRT regimens and the watch-and-wait approach following a cCR. Curiously, 94% of these patients were able to undergo salvage therapy for early tumor regrowth and with a 75% sphincter-preservation rate. Late recurrences (developing after the initial 12 months of follow-up) were observed in an additional 11% of patients. Salvage among late recurrences was possible in 91% of the cases, with sphincter preservation in 35%.[50]

When early regrowths and late recurrences are grouped together, the 5-year local recurrence rate is 68%. However, when salvage is considered in combination with the watch-and-wait strategy, the 5-year rate of local recurrence not amenable to salvage was as low as 6%. These results reinforce the importance of strict follow-up to these patients in providing optimal local disease control and immediate salvage in the event of a local recurrence (early or late).[50] It will be interesting to see whether local recurrence rates are reduced with more intensive CRT regimens with increased doses of RT and chemotherapy.

SYSTEMIC RECURRENCE

Patients with pCR are still at risk for the development of systemic recurrences. In a pooled analysis of more than 3000 patients with pCR, the distant metastases rate was 11%. Curiously, nearly 40% of this cohort ultimately received adjuvant chemotherapy.[9]

Distant metastases have been reported in 14% of patients with cCR managed nonoperatively. Ultimately, 18% of patients with local recurrences and 13% without any local recurrence were found to have metastatic disease at follow-up. Only patients with early regrowth were at risk for developing distant metastases.[50] These observations may further emphasize the opportunity for adjuvant chemotherapy in patients with cCR.

SUPPLEMENTARY DATA

Supplementary data related to this article can be found online at http://dx.doi.org/10.1016/j.hoc.2014.09.004.

REFERENCES

1. Kosinski L, Habr-Gama A, Ludwig K, et al. Shifting concepts in rectal cancer management: a review of contemporary primary rectal cancer treatment strategies. CA Cancer J Clin 2012;62:173–202.
2. Sauer R, Becker H, Hohenberger W, et al. Preoperative versus postoperative chemoradiotherapy for rectal cancer. N Engl J Med 2004;351:1731–40.
3. Kapiteijn E, Marijnen CA, Nagtegaal ID, et al. Preoperative radiotherapy combined with total mesorectal excision for resectable rectal cancer. N Engl J Med 2001;345:638–46.
4. Sauer R, Liersch T, Merkel S, et al. Preoperative versus postoperative chemoradiotherapy for locally advanced rectal cancer: results of the German CAO/ARO/AIO-94 randomized phase III trial after a median follow-up of 11 years. J Clin Oncol 2012;30:1926–33.
5. Peeters KC, van de Velde CJ, Leer JW, et al. Late side effects of short-course preoperative radiotherapy combined with total mesorectal excision for rectal cancer: increased bowel dysfunction in irradiated patients–a Dutch colorectal cancer group study. J Clin Oncol 2005;23:6199–206.
6. van Gijn W, Marijnen CA, Nagtegaal ID, et al. Preoperative radiotherapy combined with total mesorectal excision for resectable rectal cancer: 12-year follow-up of the multicentre, randomised controlled TME trial. Lancet Oncol 2011;12:575–82.
7. Bosset JF, Calais G, Mineur L, et al. Enhanced tumorocidal effect of chemotherapy with preoperative radiotherapy for rectal cancer: preliminary results–EORTC 22921. J Clin Oncol 2005;23:5620–7.
8. Schrag D, Weiser MR, Goodman KA, et al. Neoadjuvant FOLFOX-bev, without radiation, for locally advanced rectal cancer. J Clin Oncol 2010;28(Suppl) [abstract: 3511].
9. Maas M, Nelemans PJ, Valentini V, et al. Long-term outcome in patients with a pathological complete response after chemoradiation for rectal cancer: a pooled analysis of individual patient data. Lancet Oncol 2010;11:835–44.
10. Smith FM, Waldron D, Winter DC. Rectum-conserving surgery in the era of chemoradiotherapy. Br J Surg 2010;97:1752–64.
11. Habr-Gama A, Perez RO. Non-operative management of rectal cancer after neoadjuvant chemoradiation. Br J Surg 2009;96:125–7.
12. Perez RO, Habr-Gama A, Gama-Rodrigues J, et al. Accuracy of positron emission tomography/computed tomography and clinical assessment in the detection of complete rectal tumor regression after neoadjuvant chemoradiation: long-term results of a prospective trial (National Clinical Trial 00254683). Cancer 2012;118:3501–11.
13. Sanghera P, Wong DW, McConkey CC, et al. Chemoradiotherapy for rectal cancer: an updated analysis of factors affecting pathological response. Clin Oncol (R Coll Radiol) 2008;20:176–83.
14. Garcia-Aguilar J, Shi Q, Thomas CR Jr, et al. A phase II trial of neoadjuvant chemoradiation and local excision for T2N0 rectal cancer: preliminary results of the ACOSOG Z6041 trial. Ann Surg Oncol 2012;19:384–91.
15. Lezoche E, Baldarelli M, Lezoche G, et al. Randomized clinical trial of endoluminal locoregional resection versus laparoscopic total mesorectal excision for T2 rectal cancer after neoadjuvant therapy. Br J Surg 2012;99:1211–8.
16. Habr-Gama A, Perez RO, Nadalin W, et al. Operative versus nonoperative treatment for stage 0 distal rectal cancer following chemoradiation therapy: long-term results. Ann Surg 2004;240:711–7 [discussion: 717–8].

17. Radu C, Berglund A, Pahlman L, et al. Short-course preoperative radiotherapy with delayed surgery in rectal cancer - a retrospective study. Radiother Oncol 2008;87:343-9.
18. Bujko K, Nowacki MP, Nasierowska-Guttmejer A, et al. Long-term results of a randomized trial comparing preoperative short-course radiotherapy with preoperative conventionally fractionated chemoradiation for rectal cancer. Br J Surg 2006;93: 1215-23.
19. Habr-Gama A, Perez RO, Sabbaga J, et al. Increasing the rates of complete response to neoadjuvant chemoradiotherapy for distal rectal cancer: results of a prospective study using additional chemotherapy during the resting period. Dis Colon Rectum 2009;52:1927-34.
20. Habr-Gama A, Sabbaga J, Gama-Rodrigues J, et al. Watch and wait approach following extended neoadjuvant chemoradiation for distal rectal cancer: are we getting closer to anal cancer management? Dis Colon Rectum 2013;56:1109-17.
21. Hiotis SP, Weber SM, Cohen AM, et al. Assessing the predictive value of clinical complete response to neoadjuvant therapy for rectal cancer: an analysis of 488 patients. J Am Coll Surg 2002;194:131-5 [discussion: 135-6].
22. Smith FM, Chang KH, Sheahan K, et al. The surgical significance of residual mucosal abnormalities in rectal cancer following neoadjuvant chemoradiotherapy. Br J Surg 2012;99:993-1001.
23. Kalady MF, de Campos-Lobato LF, Stocchi L, et al. Predictive factors of pathologic complete response after neoadjuvant chemoradiation for rectal cancer. Ann Surg 2009;250:582-9.
24. Tulchinsky H, Shmueli E, Figer A, et al. An interval >7 weeks between neoadjuvant therapy and surgery improves pathologic complete response and disease-free survival in patients with locally advanced rectal cancer. Ann Surg Oncol 2008;15:2661-7.
25. Francois Y, Nemoz CJ, Baulieux J, et al. Influence of the interval between preoperative radiation therapy and surgery on downstaging and on the rate of sphincter-sparing surgery for rectal cancer: the Lyon R90-01 randomized trial. J Clin Oncol 1999;17:2396.
26. Evans J, Tait D, Swift I, et al. Timing of surgery following preoperative therapy in rectal cancer: the need for a prospective randomized trial? Dis Colon Rectum 2011;54:1251-9.
27. Perez RO, Habr-Gama A, Sao Juliao GP, et al. Optimal timing for assessment of tumor response to neoadjuvant chemoradiation in patients with rectal cancer: do all patients benefit from waiting longer than 6 weeks? Int J Radiat Oncol Biol Phys 2012;84:1159-65.
28. Habr-Gama A, de Souza PM, Ribeiro U Jr, et al. Low rectal cancer: impact of radiation and chemotherapy on surgical treatment. Dis Colon Rectum 1998;41: 1087-96.
29. Habr-Gama A, Perez RO, Wynn G, et al. Complete clinical response after neoadjuvant chemoradiation therapy for distal rectal cancer: characterization of clinical and endoscopic findings for standardization. Dis Colon Rectum 2010; 53:1692-8.
30. Duldulao MP, Lee W, Streja L, et al. Distribution of residual cancer cells in the bowel wall after neoadjuvant chemoradiation in patients with rectal cancer. Dis Colon Rectum 2013;56:142-9.
31. Perez RO, Habr-Gama A, Pereira GV, et al. Role of biopsies in patients with residual rectal cancer following neoadjuvant chemoradiation after downsizing: can they rule out persisting cancer? Colorectal Dis 2012;14:714-20.

32. Mignanelli ED, de Campos-Lobato LF, Stocchi L, et al. Downstaging after chemo-radiotherapy for locally advanced rectal cancer: is there more (tumor) than meets the eye? Dis Colon Rectum 2010;53:251–6.

33. Bujko K, Nowacki MP, Nasierowska-Guttmejer A, et al. Prediction of mesorectal nodal metastases after chemoradiation for rectal cancer: results of a rando-mised trial: implication for subsequent local excision. Radiother Oncol 2005; 76:234–40.

34. Kim DW, Kim DY, Kim TH, et al. Is T classification still correlated with lymph node status after preoperative chemoradiotherapy for rectal cancer? Cancer 2006;106: 1694–700.

35. Lambregts DM, Beets GL, Maas M, et al. Accuracy of gadofosveset-enhanced MRI for nodal staging and restaging in rectal cancer. Ann Surg 2011;253: 539–45.

36. Marks JH, Valsdottir EB, DeNittis A, et al. Transanal endoscopic microsurgery for the treatment of rectal cancer: comparison of wound complication rates with and without neoadjuvant radiation therapy. Surg Endosc 2009;23:1081–7.

37. Perez RO, Habr-Gama A, Sao Juliao GP, et al. Transanal endoscopic microsur-gery for residual rectal cancer after neoadjuvant chemoradiation therapy is asso-ciated with significant immediate pain and hospital readmission rates. Dis Colon Rectum 2011;54:545–51.

38. Perez RO, Habr-Gama A, Lynn PB, et al. Transanal endoscopic microsurgery for residual rectal cancer (ypT0-2) following neoadjuvant chemoradiation therapy: another word of caution. Dis Colon Rectum 2013;56:6–13.

39. Bujko K, Richter P, Kolodziejczyk M, et al. Preoperative radiotherapy and local excision of rectal cancer with immediate radical re-operation for poor responders. Radiother Oncol 2009;92:195–201.

40. Lambregts DM, Vandecaveye V, Barbaro B, et al. Diffusion-weighted MRI for se-lection of complete responders after chemoradiation for locally advanced rectal cancer: a multicenter study. Ann Surg Oncol 2011;18:2224–31.

41. Restivo A, Zorcolo L, Cocco IM, et al. Elevated CEA levels and low distance of the tumor from the anal verge are predictors of incomplete response to chemoradia-tion in patients with rectal cancer. Ann Surg Oncol 2013;20:864–71.

42. Patel UB, Taylor F, Blomqvist L, et al. Magnetic resonance imaging-detected tumor response for locally advanced rectal cancer predicts survival outcomes: MERCURY experience. J Clin Oncol 2011;29:3753–60.

43. Habr-Gama A, Perez RO, Nadalin W, et al. Long-term results of preoperative che-moradiation for distal rectal cancer correlation between final stage and survival. J Gastrointest Surg 2005;9:90–9 [discussion: 99–101].

44. Martellucci J, Scheiterle M, Lorenzi B, et al. Accuracy of transrectal ultrasound after preoperative radiochemotherapy compared to computed tomography and magnetic resonance in locally advanced rectal cancer. Int J Colorectal Dis 2012;27:967–73.

45. Murad-Regadas SM, Regadas FS, Rodrigues LV, et al. Criteria for three-dimensional anorectal ultrasound assessment of response to chemoradiotherapy in rectal cancer patients. Colorectal Dis 2011;13:1344–50.

46. Kristiansen C, Loft A, Berthelsen AK, et al. PET/CT and histopathologic response to preoperative chemoradiation therapy in locally advanced rectal cancer. Dis Colon Rectum 2008;51:21–5.

47. Das P, Skibber JM, Rodriguez-Bigas MA, et al. Predictors of tumor response and downstaging in patients who receive preoperative chemoradiation for rectal cancer. Cancer 2007;109:1750–5.

48. Perez RO, Sao Juliao GP, Habr-Gama A, et al. The role of carcinoembriogenic antigen in predicting response and survival to neoadjuvant chemoradiotherapy for distal rectal cancer. Dis Colon Rectum 2009;52:1137–43.
49. Kim CW, Yu CS, Yang SS, et al. Clinical significance of pre- to post-chemoradiotherapy s-CEA reduction ratio in rectal cancer patients treated with preoperative chemoradiotherapy and curative resection. Ann Surg Oncol 2011; 18:3271–7.
50. Habr-Gama A, Gama-Rodrigues J, Sao Juliao GP, et al. Local recurrence after complete clinical response and watch and wait in rectal cancer after neoadjuvant chemoradiation: impact of salvage therapy on local disease control. Int J Radiat Oncol Biol Phys 2014;88:822–8.

A Critical Look at Local-Regional Management of Peritoneal Metastasis

Carlos H.F. Chan, MD, PhD[a], James C. Cusack, MD[a], David P. Ryan, MD[b],*

KEYWORDS

- Colorectal cancer • Carcinomatosis • Cytoreductive surgery
- Hyperthermic intraperitoneal chemotherapy • Systemic chemotherapy

KEY POINTS

- For patients with stage IV colorectal cancer, the presence of peritoneal metastases is a poor prognostic feature.
- Despite the improvement in systemic therapy, long-term survival remains poor for patients with peritoneal carcinomatosis.
- Cytoreductive surgery (CRS) and hyperthermic intraperitoneal chemotherapy (HIPEC) can be associated with long-term survival in patients who have limited peritoneal disease, particularly those who can have complete cytoreduction.
- Whether the possible benefit of CRS and HIPEC is from the surgical resection of all disease or the combination of CRS and HIPEC remains unclear.

INTRODUCTION

Colorectal cancer is the third most common cancer and cause of cancer-related deaths in the United States.[1] Approximately 40% and 20% of patients have regional and distant metastases at the time of diagnosis, respectively.[1] Approximately 4% to 5% of patients have synchronous peritoneal metastasis at the initial presentation, accounting for 20% to 25% of all stage IV disease.[2,3] Another 3% to 5% of patients develop metachronous peritoneal metastasis after curative resection of stage I through III diseases.[2,4] Although the incidence of developing peritoneal metastasis in patients who initially presented with liver metastasis alone is not well defined, 10% to 20% of patients with metastatic disease will have synchronous and/or

[a] Division of Surgical Oncology, Massachusetts General Hospital Cancer Center, Yawkey 7B, 55 Fruit Street, Boston, MA 02114, USA; [b] Division of Medical Oncology, Massachusetts General Hospital Cancer Center, Yawkey 7B, 55 Fruit Street, Boston, MA 02114, USA
* Corresponding author.
E-mail address: DPRYAN@mgh.harvard.edu

Hematol Oncol Clin N Am 29 (2015) 153–158
http://dx.doi.org/10.1016/j.hoc.2014.09.006
0889-8588/15/$ – see front matter © 2015 Elsevier Inc. All rights reserved.

metachronous peritoneal disease.[5,6] Based on a large study pooling 2101 patients from the 2 North Central Cancer Treatment Group (NCCTG) N9741 and N9841 trials, 17% of patients with stage IV diseases had peritoneal metastases, whereas 2% of cases had isolated peritoneal metastases.[7]

Peritoneal metastasis of colorectal origin poses a significant clinical challenge. Historically, when 5-fluorouracil (5-FU) was the only available treatment for colorectal cancer, the median overall survival was 6 to 9 months[8] and the 5-year overall survival was 1%.[9] Before the availability of multiple anticancer agents, investigators used cytoreductive surgery and hyperthermic intraperitoneal chemotherapy (CRS-HIPEC) for peritoneal metastasis of colorectal origin and reported a median survival for treated patients of between 12.8 to 60.1 months and a 5-year survival rate of 11% to 48%.[10] Some treatment centers have also included early postoperative intraperitoneal chemotherapy (EPIC) as part of the regimen.[11] With the addition of multiple anticancer agents, the median overall survival for patients with metastatic colon cancer is approximately 2 years, and 20% of patients will live for 5 years or longer.[7,12] Given the improvement of current systemic treatment with various targeted therapies, the role of CRS-HIPEC and EPIC compared with systemic chemotherapy is debated.

MANAGEMENT WITH SYSTEMIC CHEMOTHERAPY ALONE

With the addition of oxaliplatin, irinotecan, and biologics including bevacizumab, cetuximab and panitumumab, the overall survival of patients with metastatic disease has notably increased. However, the impact of peritoneal metastasis on the treatment efficacy and overall survival is not clearly defined for several reasons: (1) most of the published series mixed all of the patients with stage IV disease, (2) peritoneal metastases appear in less than 20% of patients with stage IV, and (3) peritoneal metastases are often associated with other sites of metastasis. Nevertheless, a large study specifically examined the survival of patients with peritoneal metastasis by pooling 2101 with stage IV disease from the 2 NCCTG N9741 and N9841 trials.[7] In this study, 364 patients (17%) had peritoneal metastasis and 1731 patients (83%) had nonperitoneal metastasis.[7] No significant difference was seen between the groups in terms of age, gender, Eastern Cooperative Oncology Group status, and chemotherapeutic agents used. The only statistically significant differences were a higher number of metastatic sites and a lower number of associated liver and lung metastasis in patients with peritoneal metastasis.[7] Patients with peritoneal metastasis had a lower median overall survival despite having a lower incidence of synchronous liver or lung metastasis: 12.7 versus 17.6 months in patients without peritoneal metastasis. The 5-year survival rate was 4% for patients with peritoneal metastasis versus 6% for patients without peritoneal metastasis. Among patients treated with first-line FOLFOX (5-FU, leucovorin, oxaliplatin), those with peritoneal metastasis had a median overall survival of 15.7 versus 20.9 months in those without peritoneal metastasis. Although many patients in these studies were accrued before the benefit of second-line bevacizumab and the correct use of cetuximab and panitumumab in patients with *KRAS* wild-type tumors were understood, the results highlight the poor prognosis for patients with peritoneal metastases.

MANAGEMENT WITH CYTOREDUCTIVE SURGERY, HYPERTHERMIC INTRAPERITONEAL CHEMOTHERAPY, AND EARLY POSTOPERATIVE INTRAPERITONEAL CHEMOTHERAPY

CRS-HIPEC was introduced as a treatment option for peritoneal carcinomatosis disseminated from colorectal cancer in 1990s.[13] It involves surgical removal of all peritoneal surface tumors and involved organs. At the time of surgery, the abdominal cavity is fully examined to determine the extent of disease using the peritoneal carcinomatosis index (PCI) scoring system. PCI is calculated based on the number of regions involved and the maximum size of tumor deposits in each region; scores range from 0 to 36. The completeness of cytoreduction is defined as removal of all tumors more than 2.5 mm in maximum diameter (CC0 and CC1). CC0 indicates no residual disease, whereas CC2 indicates residual tumors more than or equal to 2.5 mm in size. After CRS, all intraperitoneal surfaces are exposed to heated chemotherapy. The chemotherapeutic agents, incubating temperature, duration of exposure, and techniques used vary among centers.

EPIC with various chemotherapeutic agents has also been used in some centers. In a multi-institutional registry study, Glehen and colleagues[11] collected data on 506 patients who underwent CRS-HIPEC with or without EPIC from 28 institutions. Most of these patients had adenocarcinoma of colorectal origin, except 3% of the cohort who had an unknown primary site. Complete cytoreduction could be achieved in 75% of patients (CC0: N = 271, CC1: N = 106). HIPEC and EPIC were performed in 76% and 46% of patients, respectively; 22% of patients had both HIPEC and EPIC. HIPEC was commonly performed with mitomycin C (71%). Other regimens included mitomycin C with cisplatin (13%) and oxaliplatin (8%). The regimen of 5-FU with or without mitomycin C (96%) was commonly used for EPIC. With a median follow-up of 53 months, the median overall survival was 19.2 months and the overall 1-, 3-, and 5-year survival rates were 72%, 39%, and 19%, respectively. In patients with no residual disease after cytoreduction (ie, CC0) or low burden of disease at initial exploration, the median overall survival could be as high as 32.4 or 34.8 months, respectively. Notably, 54% of patients received preoperative chemotherapy, but no difference in overall survival was seen. In contrast, patients who received postoperative 5-FU–based chemotherapy (40%) had a better median overall survival (25.2 vs 15.6 months; $P =$ .021). However, no statistically significant difference was seen among patients treated with HIPEC, EPIC, or combined HIPEC/EPIC (overall survival, 19.2, 19.2, and 21.6 months, respectively). Given the variability among different centers, it was difficult to conclude which regional therapy protocol was superior. Nonetheless, a consensus statement was published in 2006 to standardize the CRS-HIPEC treatment protocol and to establish patient selection criteria based on existing evidence.[14]

In a retrospective multi-institutional analysis, Elias and colleagues[15] reviewed 523 patients who underwent CRS-HIPEC/EPIC for colorectal peritoneal metastasis in 23 institutions between 1990 and 2007; 14% of these patients had an unknown primary site. The median overall survival reached 30.1 months and the 5-year survival rate was 27%. The apparent higher survival may have been influenced by better patient selection. In this study, 84% of patients had CC0 level of cytoreduction (vs 54% in the study reported by Glehen and colleagues[11]). In addition, 65% of patients had limited disease, indicated by a PCI of 12 or less (vs 34% in the study reported by Glehen and colleagues[11]). In fact, Glehen and colleagues[11] also showed similar survival when the completeness of cytoreduction and low PCI were considered. In a systematic review and meta-analysis of all the CRS-HIPEC studies between 1995 and 2009, Chua and colleagues[16] showed that the median overall survival of patients with complete cytoreduction (N = 722) was 33 months (range, 20–63 months) and the median 5-year survival rate was 43% (range, 20%–51%). In contrast, patients with incomplete cytoreduction had a much poorer outcome, with a median overall survival of only 8 months (range, 4–17 months) and a 5-year survival rate of 0%. These findings again showed that proper patient selection might be the key to success in CRS-HIPEC.

However, these retrospective studies did not address an important question. Given the fact that more than half of the patients received perioperative chemotherapy, the question remains as to whether CRS-HIPEC added a survival benefit. Verwaal and colleagues[17] tested this treatment paradigm on peritoneal metastasis of colorectal cancer in a prospective randomized controlled trial in the Netherlands between 1998 and 2001. This trial randomly assigned 105 patients with isolated peritoneal metastasis of colorectal origin into 2 treatment groups: standard treatment with systemic 5-FU/leucovorin alone (N = 51) and CRS-HIPEC followed by systemic 5-FU/leucovorin (N = 54). With a median follow-up of 21.6 months, this trial showed a survival difference in favor of CRS-HIPEC followed by systemic treatment (22.4 vs 12.6 months in the systemic treatment alone arm; P = .032). With a median follow-up of 8 years, the median disease-specific survival was 22.2 months in the CRS-HIPEC treatment arm, versus 12.6 months in the standard treatment arm.[18] However, with the longer follow-up, 4 patients remained alive in the standard treatment group (2 with disease and 2 without disease) and 5 remained alive in the CRS-HIPEC group (2 with disease and 3 without disease). This trial also demonstrated that complete cytoreduction (ie, residual tumor size<2.5 mm) and limited peritoneal disease were significant prognostic factors in the CRS-HIPEC group.[17]

Although this trial showed an improvement in overall survival associated with CRS-HIPEC followed by systemic treatment, the study was limited by several factors. First, the validity of the trial was compromised by including 18 appendiceal cancers (17% of patient population). Appendiceal mucinous neoplasms and appendiceal adenocarcinomas are sometimes difficult to differentiate on pathologic analysis. The natural history of appendiceal cancers varies widely, and inclusion of any patients with appendiceal cancer as opposed to colorectal adenocarcinoma can compromise the results of the study. Second, although an incremental survival benefit of 10 months was shown in the CRS-HIPEC group, the added benefit may not be equivalent to that associated with modern systemic chemotherapeutic regimens including oxaliplatin or irinotecan. Third, although advocates of CRS-HIPEC[18] emphasize the long-term survival seen in surgical series, the long-term survival in the control arm of the one randomized study was equivalent to the treatment arm. Lastly, whether the added survival benefit was a result of CRS, HIPEC, or both was unclear.

Surgically rendering patients free of all disease is associated with cure for patients with isolated liver or lung metastases. It is reasonable to assume that some patients who have isolated and limited peritoneal metastases that can be resected will experience a cure. Although the surgical series suggest that this may be the case, the independent effects of CRS from HIPEC are difficult to tease out because these treatments are almost always administered together. To address the true efficacy of HIPEC alone, a French multicenter, randomized, controlled trial (Prodige 7) is currently underway.[19] This trial has the goal of randomizing 280 patients with complete cytoreduction into 2 arms (HIPEC using intraperitoneal oxaliplatin and intravenous 5-FU/leucovorin over 30 minutes at a minimum of 42C vs no HIPEC). The primary endpoint is 3- and 5-year overall survival. Although most of the existing data on CRS-HIPEC are based on the use of mitomycin C, the results from this trial may shed some light on whether HIPEC using intraperitoneal oxaliplatin with intravenous 5-FU/leucovorin improves survival. However, this trial will not be able to address the potential added benefit of HIPEC with mitomycin C to CRS in the existing published data. Unfortunately, a multicenter randomized controlled trial addressing this specific question, conducted by Walter Reed Army Medical Center and the American College of Surgeons,[20] was closed prematurely because of a poor accrual.

HIGH MORBIDITY AND MORTALITY RATES ASSOCIATED WITH LOCAL-REGIONAL THERAPY

Postoperative mortality and morbidity are significant concerns in patients treated with CRS-HIPEC compared with those receiving systemic chemotherapy alone. The postoperative mortality rate associated with CRS-HIPEC ranges from 0% to 12% in various surgical series,[10] and is commonly quoted as 3% to 4% based on the 2 largest studies.[11,15] Septic shock, respiratory complications, pulmonary embolism, hematologic toxicity, cerebral stroke, peritonitis, and renal insufficiency were reported as causes of death in these 2 series.[11,15] The postoperative morbidity rate of CRS-HIPEC has been reported to be between 23.0% and 55.6% in various surgical series.[10] Grade 3–4 complications were reported in 23% to 31% of patients in the 2 large series.[11,15] Digestive fistulas were reported in 8% to 9% of patients in both large series. Hematologic toxicity was reported between 2% and 12% of patients in these series. The latter discrepancy may have been related to the chemotherapy agent used. In the French multicentric study reported by Elias and colleagues,[15] 45% of patients had oxaliplatin-based HIPEC and 55% had mitomycin C-based HIPEC, whereas 8%, 13% and 71% of patients had oxaliplatin-, cisplatin- and mitomycin C-based HIPEC, respectively, in the study reported by Glehen and colleagues.[11] However, further studies will be required to evaluate this potential association. The other grade 3–4 complications include infectious complications (systemic sepsis, line sepsis, intra-abdominal abscess/peritonitis, pulmonary infection), postoperative bleeding, respiratory distress, pulmonary embolism, urinary fistula, and bowel obstruction.[11,15]

SUMMARY AND FUTURE DIRECTION

For patients with stage IV colorectal cancer, the presence of peritoneal metastases is a poor prognostic feature. Despite the improvement in systemic therapy, long-term survival remains poor for patients with peritoneal carcinomatosis. Surgical series suggest that CRS and HIPEC can be associated with long-term survival in patients who have limited peritoneal disease, particularly those who can have complete cytoreduction. Whether the possible benefit of CRS and HIPEC is from the surgical resection of all disease or the combination of CRS and HIPEC remains unclear. Further clinical trials are needed to clarity the role of surgery and intraperitoneal chemotherapy in patients with peritoneal carcinomatosis.

REFERENCES

1. Siegel R, Naishadham D, Jemal A. Cancer statistics, 2013. CA Cancer J Clin 2013;63:11–30.
2. Segelman J, Granath F, Holm T, et al. Incidence, prevalence and risk factors for peritoneal carcinomatosis from colorectal cancer. Br J Surg 2012;99:699–705.
3. Lemmens VE, Klaver YL, Verwaal VJ, et al. Predictors and survival of synchronous peritoneal carcinomatosis of colorectal origin: a population-based study. Int J Cancer 2011;128:2717–25.
4. van Gestel YR, Thomassen I, Lemmens VE, et al. Metachronous peritoneal carcinomatosis after curative treatment of colorectal cancer. Eur J Surg Oncol 2013; 40(8):963–9.
5. Sjo OH, Berg M, Merok MA, et al. Peritoneal carcinomatosis of colon cancer origin: highest incidence in women and in patients with right-sided tumors. J Surg Oncol 2011;104:792–7.
6. Kerscher AG, Chua TC, Gasser M, et al. Impact of peritoneal carcinomatosis in the disease history of colorectal cancer management: a longitudinal experience of 2406 patients over two decades. Br J Cancer 2013;108:1432–9.
7. Franko J, Shi Q, Goldman CD, et al. Treatment of colorectal peritoneal carcinomatosis with systemic chemotherapy: a pooled analysis of north central cancer treatment group phase III trials N9741 and N9841. J Clin Oncol 2012;30:263–7.

8. Koppe MJ, Boerman OC, Oyen WJG, et al. Peritoneal carcinomatosis of colorectal origin: incidence and current treatment strategies. Ann Surg 2006;243: 212–22.
9. Dy GK, Hobday TJ, Nelson G, et al. Long-term survivors of metastatic colorectal cancer treated with systemic chemotherapy alone: a North Central Cancer Treatment Group review of 3811 patients, N0144. Clin Colorectal Cancer 2009;8: 88–93.
10. Weber T, Roitman M, Link KH. Current status of cytoreductive surgery with hyperthermic intraperitoneal chemotherapy in patients with peritoneal carcinomatosis from colorectal cancer. Clin Colorectal Cancer 2012;11:167–76.
11. Glehen O, Kwiatkowski F, Sugarbaker PH, et al. Cytoreductive surgery combined with perioperative intraperitoneal chemotherapy for the management of peritoneal carcinomatosis from colorectal cancer: a multi-institutional study. J Clin Oncol 2004;22:3284–92.
12. Kopetz S, Chang GJ, Overman MJ, et al. Improved survival in metastatic colorectal cancer is associated with adoption of hepatic resection and improved chemotherapy. J Clin Oncol 2009;27:3677–83.
13. Sugarbaker PH. Patient selection and treatment of peritoneal carcinomatosis from colorectal and appendiceal cancer. World J Surg 1995;19:235–40.
14. Esquivel J, Sticca R, Sugarbaker P, et al. Cytoreductive surgery and hyperthermic intraperitoneal chemotherapy in the management of peritoneal surface malignancies of colonic origin: a consensus statement. Ann Surg Oncol 2006;14: 128–33.
15. Elias D, Gilly F, Boutitie F, et al. Peritoneal colorectal carcinomatosis treated with surgery and perioperative intraperitoneal chemotherapy: retrospective analysis of 523 patients from a multicentric French study. J Clin Oncol 2010;28:63–8.
16. Chua TC, Esquivel J, Pelz JOW, et al. Summary of current therapeutic option for peritoneal metastases from colorectal cancer. J Surg Oncol 2013;107:566–73.
17. Verwaal VJ, van Ruth S, de Bree E, et al. Randomized trial of cytoreduction and hyperthermic intraperitoneal chemotherapy versus systemic chemotherapy and palliative surgery in patients with peritoneal carcinomatosis of colorectal cancer. J Clin Oncol 2003;21:3737–43.
18. Verwaal VJ, Bruin S, Boot H, et al. 8-year follow-up of randomized trial: cytoreduction and hyperthermic intraperitoneal chemotherapy versus systemic chemotherapy in patients with peritoneal carcinomatosis of colorectal cancer. Ann Surg Oncol 2008;15:2426–32.
19. Elias D, Quenet F, Goere D. Current status and future directions in the treatment of peritoneal dissemination from colorectal carcinoma. Surg Oncol Clin N Am 2012;21:611–23.
20. Avital I, Brücher BL, Nissan A, et al. Randomized Clinical Trials for Colorectal Cancer Peritoneal Surface Malignancy. Surg Oncol Clin N Am 2012;21:665–88.

Index

Note: Page numbers of article titles are in **boldface** type.

http://dx.doi.org/10.1016/S0889-8588(14)00164-6
0889-8588/15/$ – see front matter

Moving?

Make sure your subscription moves with you!

To notify us of your new address, find your **Clinics Account Number** (located on your mailing label above your name), and contact customer service at:

Email: journalscustomerservice-usa@elsevier.com

800-654-2452 (subscribers in the U.S. & Canada)
314-447-8871 (subscribers outside of the U.S. & Canada)

Fax number: 314-447-8029

Elsevier Health Sciences Division
Subscription Customer Service
3251 Riverport Lane
Maryland Heights, MO 63043

*To ensure uninterrupted delivery of your subscription, please notify us at least 4 weeks in advance of move.